PEARLS OF MEDICINE

LONG CASE

Khan H

Self-publishing at KDP

Dedicated to my beloved parents, great teachers, especially Professor Nasir ud Din Azam Khan and Dr. SGN Richardson, my brilliant students, caring family, and loving friends and classmates, in particular the KMC class of 80 and the late Dr. Sarfaraz Khan alias Amir-sahib.

"And the one, who saved a life, is surely as if he had saved the whole mankind."

AL-QURAN, SURA AL-MAIDA; 5:32

CONTENTS

Title Page

Copyright

Dedication

Epigraph

Introduction

Preface

ABBREVIATIONS

INTRODUCTION TO LONG CASE   1

FORMAT OF LONG CASE   3

EXAMINATION KIT   5

HISTORY TAKING   7

PHYSICAL EXAMINATION   9

TEMPLATE OF HISTORY & PHYSICAL EXAM   12

CLERKING   17

PRESENTATION   21

DISCUSSION   23

PIT-FALLS DURING DISCUSSION   25

EXPECTATIONS OF EXAMINERS   27

PLANNING FOR PREPARATION   29

BACKGROUND KNOWLEDGE   32

COMMON LONG CASES   33

DIABETES MELLITUS   35

HYPERTENSION	61
CHRONIC LIVER DISEASE	95
CEREBROVASCULAR DISEASE	140
CHRONIC OBSTRUCTIVE PULMONARY DISEASE	236
CHRONIC KIDNEY DISEASE	256
CORONARY HEART DISEASE	300
SYSTEMIC LUPUS ERYTHEMATOSUS	336
MULTIPLE SCLEROSIS	356
BIBLIOGRAPHY	376
Acknowledgement	381
About The Author	383

INTRODUCTION

T his book is basically an aid to prepare for the long-case in clinical examinations of Internal Medicine and allied subjects. As we know, long-case is an integral component of any clinical examination and its purpose is to check whether the candidate is prepared enough to deal with the patients in a safe and logical way.

This work will help not only the students to go through their clinical exams successfully but will also be an aid for the practicing physicians.

PREFACE

Medicine is a vast subject and there are innumerable books written on its every aspect. But astonishingly the books written to guide the students to tackle through their long-case during examinations are quite a few. Undergraduate medical students in general and postgraduate in particular find minimal help in this respect while they are preparing for their final exams. This apparent gap in the publication tempted me to write on this topic.

I was thinking over it and compiling my notes and the rele-vant literature for a long time since my induction as faculty of Gomal Medical College, D.I.Khan. My colleague and friend Dr. Khadim Hussain used to motivate me to write a book and the title Pearls of Medicine was in fact suggested by him. However, it was the lockdown during COVID-19 pandemic which acted as a blessing in disguise for me and provided me an opportunity to fulfill this long awaited desire.

As a matter of fact some well-standardized postgraduate exams have excluded the long-case section from their format and have modified the short cases in such a way as to cover the skills previously tested during the long-case. It is important to note that the skills developed while prepar-ing for a long-case would certainly be helpful for those examinees as well.

This book will not only help the students and postgrads for preparation of their exams but will also help to improve the quality of care provided by the physicians in their day-to-day clinical practice.

In the initial chapters the general aspects and principles to deal with a long-case are elaborated and in the late the individual long-cases are discussed in details. Each long-case has the subheadings; Summary, Management plan, Discussion, and Land-mark trials. The student while reading the book will feel as if he was in the exam situation. This confidence of sound preparation at the back of his mind will keep him relaxed and structured in the actual exam.

If you go through this book you will come across the information which you already knew but this book will give you a new zeal to tackle your difficult patients and impos-sible-looking exams to pass. The points given at the proper places will act as aide-memoire.

The language used in this book is US English because of its simplicity and ease of spelling the words.

I hope this book will be a valuable addition to the medical knowledge. The readers are requested to enlighten the editor with their comments for improvement and rectifica-tion of deficiencies in the forthcoming editions.

The Editor
Habibullah Khan, FRCP Edin
E-mail: pearlsofmedicine@gmail.com
Twitter: @Medicinepearls

ABBREVIATIONS

ABC	Airway, Breathing, Circulation
ABGs	Arterial blood gases
A&E	Accident & Emergency
ACE-I	Angiotensin converting enzyme inhibitor
ACLS	Advanced cardiac life support
ACR	Albumin creatinine ratio
ACS	Acute coronary syndrome
ACTH	Adrenocorticotrophic hormone
AE	Acute exacerbation
AER	Albumin excretion rate
AF	Atrial fibrillation
AFP	Alpha fetoprotein
AIDS	Acquired immunodeficiency syndrome
AFP	Alpha fetoprotein
AGN	Acute glomerulonephritis
AKI	Acute kidney injury
ALP	Alkaline phosphatase
ANA	Anti-nuclear antibodies
ANCA	Anti-neutrophil cytoplasmic antibodies
ARB	Angiotensin receptor blocker
AS	Aortic stenosis
AVF	Arteriovenous fistula
AZA	Azathioprine
BMI	Body mass index
BP	Blood pressure
BUN	Blood urea nitrogen
CABG	Coronary artery bypass graft
CAPD	Continuous ambulatory peritoneal dialysis
CCB	Calcium channel blocker
CCF	Congestive cardiac failure
CCU	Cardiac care unit
CI	Confidence interval
CK	Creatinine kinase
CKD	Chronic kidney disease
CK-MB	Cardiac-specific creatinine kinase
CLD	Chronic liver disease
CMV	Cytomegalo virus
CNS	Central nervous system
COPD	Chronic obstructive pulmonary disease

CrCl	Creatinine clearance
CRP	C-Reactive proteins
C/S	Culture & Sensitivity
CSF	Cerebrospinal fluid
CT	Computerized tomography
CTA	CT angiography
CV	Cardiovascular
CVA	Cerebrovascular accident
CVD	Cerebrovascular disease
CVS	Cardiovascular system
CYC	Cyclophosphamide
DBP	Diastolic blood pressure
DKA	Diabetic ketoacidosis
DM	Diabetes mellitus
DMRD	Disease-modifying drug
DSA	Digital subtraction angiography
DVT	Deep vein thrombosis
ECG	Electrocardiogram
EPO	Erythropoietin
ER	Emergency room
ESR	Erythrocyte sedimentation rate
ESRD	End-stage renal disease
EF	Ejection fraction
ETT	Exercise tolerance test
ESA	Erythropoietin stimulating agent
EVD	Extra ventricular drainage
EVL	Endoscopic variceal ligation
FBC	Full blood count
FBS	Fasting blood sugar
FDA	Food and Drugs Administration
FEV1	Forced expiratory volume in first second
FFP	Fresh frozen plasma
FVC	Forced vital capacity
GCS	Glasgow Coma Scale
GERD	Gastro-esophageal reflux disease
GFR	Glomerular filtration rate
GI	Gastro-intestinal
GLP	Glucagon-like peptide
GN	Glomerulonephritis
GP	General Practitioner
GPE	General physical examination
GTN	Glyceryl trinitrate

GTT	Glucose tolerance test
H&P	History & physical examination
HbA1c	Glycated hemoglobin
HBV	Hepatitis B virus
HCC	Hepatocellular carcinoma
HCM	Hypertrophic cardiomyopathy
HCQ	Hydroxy chloroquine
HCT	Hydrochlorothiazide
HCV	Hepatitis C virus
HD	Hemodialysis
HDU	High dependency unit
HDV	Hepatitis D virus
HDL	High-density lipoprotein
HE	Hepatic encephalopathy
HIV	Human immunodeficiency virus
HRT	Hormone replacement therapy
HT	Hypertension
ICA	Internal carotid artery
ICS	Inhaled corticosteroids
ICP	Intracranial pressure
ICU	Intensive care unit
IFN	Interferon
IGT	Impaired glucose tolerance
IHD	Ischemic heart disease
INO	Internuclear ophthalmoplegia
INR	International normalized ratio
IPD	Intermittent peritoneal dialysis
IVU	Intravenous urography
JVP	Jugular venous pressure
LABA	Long-acting beta-2 agonists
LAMA	Long-acting muscarinic antagonist
LDL	Low-density lipoprotein
LFTs	Liver function tests
LMN	Lower motor neuron
LMWH	Low molecular weight heparin
LN	Lupus nephritis
LP	Lumber puncture
LTOT	Long-term oxygen therapy
LVF	Left ventricular failure
MBD	Mineral bone disease
MCA	Middle cerebral artery
MCTD	Mixed connective tissue disease

MI	Myocardial infarction
MPI	Myocardial perfusion imaging
MR	Mitral regurgitation
MMF	Mycophenolate mofetil
MRA	Magnetic resonance angiography
MRC	Medical Research Council
MRI	Magnetic resonance imaging
MS	Multiple sclerosis
MSU	Mid-stream urine
MT	Mechanical thrombectomy
MTX	Methotrexate
NCCT	Non-contract CT scan
NG	Nasogastric
NOAC	Non-vitamin K oral anticoagulant
NODAT	New onset diabetes after transplant
NPO	Nil per oral
NSAID	Non-steroidal anti-inflammatory drug
NVAF	Nonvalvular atrial fibrillation
OCP	Oral contraceptive pill
OGD	Esophago-gastro-duodenoscopy
PAH	Pulmonary artery hypertension
PaO2	Plasma arterial oxygen saturation
PCI	Percutaneous coronary intervention
PCR	Polymerase chain reaction
PD	Peritoneal dialysis
PFO	Patent foramen ovale
PIH	Pregnancy induced hypertension
PKD	Polycystic kidney disease
PP	Post-prandial
PPI	Proton pump inhibitor
PSE	Portosystemic encephalopathy
PT	Prothrombin time
PTCA	Percutaneous transluminal coronary angioplasty
PTLD	Post-transplant lymphoproliferative disorder
PTH	Parathyroid hormone
QoL	Quality of life
RA	Rheumatoid arthritis
RAS	Renal artery stenosis
RBS	Random blood sugar
RCT	Randomized controlled trial
RFTs	Renal function tests
RR	Relative risk

RRT	Renal replacement therapy
SAAG	Serum ascetic-fluid albumin gradient
SAH	Subarachnoid hemorrhage
SaO_2	Arterial Oxygen saturation
SBP	Subacute bacterial peritonitis
SK	Streptokinase
SLE	Systemic lupus erythematosus
SOB	Shortness of breath
SOL	Space occupying lesion
STEMI	ST-elevation myocardial infarction
TAC	Tacrolimus
TACE	Transarterial chemo-embolization
TB	Tuberculosis
T2D	Type 2 diabetes mellitus
TIA	Transient ischemic attack
TIPS	Transjugular intrahepatic portosystemic shunt
TLC	Total leucocyte count
t-PA	Tissue plasminogen activator
TSAT	Transferrin saturation
U&Es	Urea and electrolytes
UMN	Upper motor neuron
USG	Ultrasonography
VMA	Vanillyl mandelic acid
WHO	World Health Organization

INTRODUCTION TO LONG CASE

L ong-case is an integral component of any clinical examination. Its purpose is to check whether the candidate is prepared to deal with patients especially those who get admitted to the hospital.

Although long-case constitutes a major part of almost all clinical examinations, yet it is given least importance by the candidates.

Some standard international examinations like MRCP UK has omitted the long-case from their format but instead has incorporated its theme in the form of Practical As-sessment of Clinical Examination Skills (PACES) which covers both the long and short cases. The current effort will of course help those candidates as well in preparation for their PACES.

Examination station is usually a small cabin with a patient's bed having a pillow and a blanket preferably with free space all around the bed and a trolley with items like hand sanitizer, tissue papers, gloves, etc. Disposable pins and orange sticks may also be available.

EXAMINATION STATION

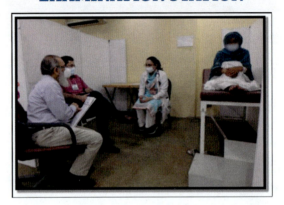

Figure 1.1: Scene of examination station during a postgrduate long-case examination.

Taken from the picture gallery at the website of the College of Physicians and Surgeons of Pakistan.

FORMAT OF LONG CASE

D uring clinical examination a patient is assigned to the candidate as a long-case. The duration of interaction is usually one hour and a pair of examiners is deployed for assessment.

In the first half; the candidate has to take a detailed history including the systemic review, perform a thorough clinical examination and make a provisional or differential diagnosis.

He has to write down the H&P and also to write a "Summary" and "Management plan" at the end of H&P.

During all this time the examiners may be observing the candidate either directly or via a video link.

In the second half; the candidate has to present the case and the examiners will discuss it with the candidate for his assessment or scoring.

The template of a typical long-case is given below. Each step will be discussed in details in the forth-coming sections.

TEMPLATE OF A LONG CASE

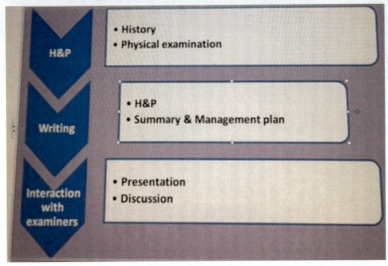

EXAMINATION KIT

Y our examination kit should have the following items in a good working condition:

- Stethoscope
- BP set
- Percussion hammer
- Pencil torch
- Orange stick (or a key with blunt edge)
- Measuring tape
- Thermometer
- Ophthalmoscope (preferably pocket size)

Optional:
- Disposable pins (May be provided in the exam)
- Red and white hat pins
- Pocket Snellen's chart
- Tuning fork 128 Htz
- Magnifying lens
- Pulse oximeter

EXAMINATION KIT

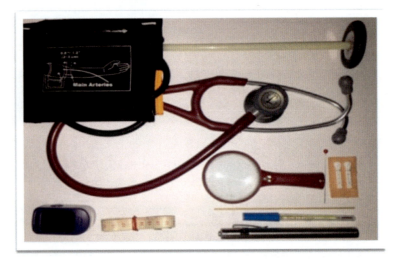

HISTORY TAKING

After introduction, preferably with a hand-shake, a detailed history is to be taken in a long-case. History taking is an art and needs a lot of practice to master it. Medical history is actually the story of a patient obtained tactfully by a professional and then written and narrated using the patient's wordings and professional terminology where appropriate.

COMPONENTS

The history includes the following sub-sections:

- Demographics
- Chief complaints
- History of present illness
- Past history
- Family history
- Drug history
- Socio-economic history
- History-based diagnosis

SYSTEMIC REVIEW

Systemic review or inquiry is performed at the end of the history by asking some prototype questions which cover most of the symptoms of diseases affecting the major organ systems. The purpose of this inquiry is to discover and fill any gaps or deficiencies in the history.

Systemic review doesn't need to be written separately; instead it is to be incorporated in the already taken history while writing it down.

The questions of systemic inquiry need to be pre-determined and can even be asked while performing the clinical examination to save the time.

HISTORY-BASED DIAGNOSIS

The history should always end-up with a "History Based Diagnosis" (HBD).

Our great teacher Professor Nasir-ud-Din Azam Khan used to stress hardly on the importance of "History Based Diagnosis" during his ward rounds. He used to say, *"It is mandatory to make the history-based diagnosis because the eyes can't see what the mind doesn't know. If you have a diagnosis in your mind, you will pick even a subtle sign, otherwise you may even miss the obvious ones."*

PHYSICAL EXAMINATION

P hysical examination should be thorough but quick and time saving. While performing physical examination do'nt forget that you have to be:

Quick: To save the time.

Fluent: To show that you have practiced thoroughly.

Tender: Taking care of the patient's comfort.

Physical Examination has two components:

- General Physical Examination
- Systemic Examination

GENERAL PHYSICAL EXAMINATION

Opening remarks:
A sentence or two stating the general condition of the patient like: stable /unstable, comfortable /short of breath, exhausted look, confused, etc.

Vital signs:

Pulse	T	BP
Resp rate	SaO_2 (if available)	

Common signs: Mark as Present (+) or Absent (0)

Anemia 0/+   Jaundice 0/+   Cyanosis 0/+   Edema 0/+

Clubbing 0/+   Koilonychia 0/+ Neck veins ↔ / ↑

Fundi, Lymph nodes, and Thyroid can also be included in the GPE if relevant.

SYSTEMIC EXAMINATION

All the systems are examined with special emphasis and detail of the one pointed-out in the history.

Along with the positive findings important negatives are also to be noted.

It includes four major systems:

- Respiratory system
- Cardiovascular system
- Abdominal system
- Nervous system

Others systems like Musculoskeletal, and Urogenital, are examined only where required.

Genitalia are routinely not examined and rectal examination is not performed during assessment exams but this to be pointed out to the examiner if required (Tell the examiner - I would normally be performing .rectal examination if allowed).

PROVISIONAL DIAGNOSIS

It is better to consider the differential diagnosis (DD) rather than a single diagnosis. It protects you from the errors in the diagnosis.

TEMPLATE OF HISTORY & PHYSICAL EXAM

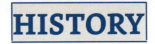

Name .... **Age/DOB** ....

Gender .... **Occupation** ....

Address (including geographic /ethnic origin)
....
....

Chief Complaints: (in a chronological order)
....
....
....

History of Present Illness: (Details of chief complaints
– a paragraph for each complaint)
....
....
....
....
....
....
....
....

....

Past History:

....

Family History:

....

Drug History:

Current ....

Previous ....

Allergies ....

Socio-economic History:

Status ....

Sources of income ....

Liabilities ....

Addiction (Tobacco /Ethanol, etc.) ....

HISTORY-BASED DIAGNOSIS

PHYSICAL EXAMINATION

GENERAL PHYSICAL EXAMINATION

General remarks:

....
....
.

| Pulse Rate | BP | Temp | Resp |

SaO_2 ((if available)

| Anemia | Jaundice | Cyanosis | Edema |
| Clubbing | Koilonychia | Neck-veins |
| L. nodes |
| Thyroid |

SYSTEMIC EXAMINATION

RESPIRATORY SYSTEM

Inspection

Palpation

Percussion

Auscultation

CARDIO-VASCULAR SYSTEM

Inspection

Palpation

Percussion

Auscultation

GASTRO-INTESTINAL SYSTEM

Inspection

Palpation

Percussion

Auscultation

NERVOUS SYSTEM

Conscious level

Memory

Speech

Cranial Nerves

Upper limbs:		Right	Left
Inspection			
Tone			
Power			
Reflexes:	Biceps		
	Triceps		
	Radial		
Lower limbs:		Right	Left

Inspection

Tone

Power

Reflexes: Knee jerk

Ankle jerk

Plantar response

OTHER

(like Musculoskeletal, Genito-urinary, etc)

PROVISIONAL DIAGNOSIS /DIFFERENCIAL DIAGNOSIS

CLERKING

O nce you have taken the detailed history and performed a thorough physical examination, sitback on the bed-side chair, take a sigh, relax for a moment and then concentrate and write it down. A template of H&P for clerking is given above for guidance.

After writing H&P, always write down a "SUMMARY" and "MANAGEMENT PLAN".

This will help in the forthcoming sessions of "PRESENTATION" and "DISCUSSION".

In the practical life also, the written H&P and SUMMARY NOTE will be helpful to quickly understand the patient's problems if someone else checks the patient notes in your absence.

SUMMARY

Summary is actually the summation of H&P and interpretation of the problem.

It must be comprehensive but concise and ideally shouldn't exceed a short paragraph. Contrary to the history, use medical terminology instead of patient's wordings in the summary.

Sequence: The summary should start with the patient's "Name", "Gender", "Age", "Occupation", and "Address" (including the ethnicity, geographic origin, or nationality).

Then it should reveal the chief complaints in a chronological order followed by important aspects of the past, family, drugs, and socio-economic history.

Then mention the positive clinical signs which have led you to the diagnosis. Important negative findings can also be mentioned.

The summary should end-up with the conclusive remarks highlighting the key issues including the diagnosis or better a differential diagnosis.

MANAGEMENT PLAN

The management plan should be presented in a narrative fashion like;

I

will ....

.

It should first address the acute problems:

- **ABC + 2S:** Symptomatic and Supportive interventions.

   Then it should address the other issues as below:

- **Investigations:** To confirm the diagnosis, rule out other important differential, and assessment for severity and cause.

   Include the routine basic investigations and specific ones relevant to the pertinent case.
- **3S:**
   Site of care: A&E, Ward, ITU, Hospice, or Home.
   Specific treatment.
   Specialty referral if needed.
- To deal with any complications.
- Assessing the response to treatment and criteria for discharge.
- Identification and Management of risk factors and patient education.
- Social /occupational /dietary needs, including life-style changes, exercise, identification bracelet, rehabilitation.
- Follow-up arrangements: Timing of outpatient visits (GP &/or Specialist),

Compliance monitoring, and preventive aspects e.g. vaccinations if applicable.

WRITING H&P, SUMMARY AND MANAGEMENT PLAN

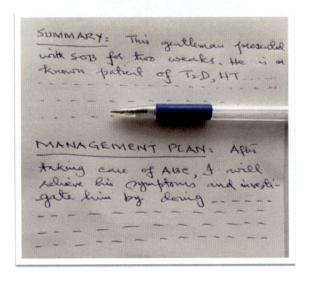

PRESENTATION

During the second half of the clinicals, the candidate will be asked to present the case. The key to success in this part of long-case is confidence. Look into the examiners eyes and present the case in a clear and organized way.

During this session imagine as if you were presenting the case to your senior colleague or your consultant in a routine ward round.

Keep the time of your presentation a bit short to leave sufficient time for discussion. If you are getting behind, the examiners may interrupt you and that may have negative impact on your flow of thoughts. Normally it should be 10-15 minutes.

OPENING QUESTION

The examiners will usually require a brief summary of the case but at times they may ask you to narrate the full H&P findings. This can be judged from the pattern of their opening question.

The common opening questions are:

- Please tell us about your patient?
- Please present your case?

- What is your diagnosis? And which features in the H&P lead you to this diagnosis?
- What is your diagnosis or differential diagnosis?

OPENING STATEMENT

I examined Mr. .... (Name), Age, Gender, Occupation, Address.

He presented with .... (Chief complaints with brief description).

ORDER OF PRESENTATION

- Chief complaints in a chronological order. Followed by any other important finding in the history.
- All positive and important negative signs on clinical examination.
- Ending-up with conclusive remarks pointing to the important issues including the diagnosis or preferably the differential diagnosis.

DISCUSSION

A fter presentation, the examiners will discuss the patient with the candidate in detail. Discussion will mostly revolves around the "assessment" and "management" issues. The examiners expect and try to confirm that the candidate should be up-to-date regarding the latest research in the relevant field.

The examiners will often ask at some stage about the prognosis of the case under discussion as well.

They may sometimes ask you to elicit or demonstrate some of the clinical signs during this part of examination to check your clinical skills.

Always give due attention to both the examiners because the one who is asking questions may not be actually marking you while the silent by-stander of the pair may be the one responsible for your scoring. A pleasant look with a light smile may be sufficient to keep him on board on your side.

During discussion the examiners will try to determine whether you are a safe doctor, and your knowledge, clinical skills, power of interpretation, and style of presentation are up to the for a consultant level.

Your presentation has created certain impression and

the examiners are now trying to validate that impression. Your response during can up-grade or down-grade your score.

In most clinical exams a printed proforma is given to both the examiners to evaluate the various clinical skills as a numerical value. Result of one aspect doesn't interfere the other, so always look forwards and forget about your performance a moment ago.

ASSESSMENT ISSUES

These include:

- Investigations to confirm the diagnosis.
- Investigations to rule-out the important differential diagnoses.
- Investigations for assessment of severity and cause.
- Investigations for complications

MANAGEMENT ISSUES

Acute Management:

ABC + 2S (Supportive and Symptomatic interventions).

Management of chronic disease:

Including its latest treatments.

Other aspects:

Social, psychological, occupational, and preventive.

T he examiners may ask you to clarify certain points in the history.

Don't consider this as something to downgrade you. It is just to check your knowledge and skills.

To prepare for this question you should master the description of symptoms as given in the first few pages of each system in the "clinical methods".

Answer briefly and elaborate the points as desired by the examiner, clarifying in a logical way.

Sometimes your findings may be challenged by the examiners.

Don't get annoyed or confused. Just lightly explain the basis for your findings in a cool manner and tactfully consider the alternative as pointed-out by the examiner.

If you had some clear-cut mistake or deficiency.

Nothing to worry, rather handle the situation smoothly and tactfully.

Do not bluff the examiners as it can be catastrophic,

while a gentle confession will resolve the issue.

Go ahead with the new findings or situation and discuss the relevance of these and its management as required.

Up to date knowledge.

Latest research in the relevant field is expected from the candidate during discussion. You must be familiar with the "Land-mark trials" and "Clinical Practice Guidelines" as issued by the reputed international bodies from time to time.

Some of the top class resources are:

Medscape: http://www.medscape.com
UpToDate: http://www.uptodate.com

Both are rich resources for the latest research and knowledge in Medicine. UpToDate is by purchase of subscription while Medscape is totally free.

You must be regularly attending the Journal clubs and must have subscribed for one of the medical journals of international repute, like BMJ, NEJM. Lancet, at least online (can be obtained free).

EXPECTATIONS OF EXAMINERS

T he examiners expect from the candidate that he/ she should be academically sound and able to:

- Take and present the history in a systematic and logical way.
- Perform the physical examination in a focused and professional way.
- Establish the correct facts from the history and elicit the relevant findings from the examination.
- Suggest appropriate investigations to establish the diagnosis and to rule-out the relevant differential diagnoses.
- Suggest appropriate management strategies for the emergency and the chronic problems.
- Present the case in clear and organized way.
- Communicate with the examiners in a clear, bold, and organized way - like a consultant.
- Must have an up-to-date knowledge.

Remember - when you are going very well, the examiners may pose more difficult questions or situations to score you high. Don't get annoyed or dis-hearted in such a situation. Difficult questions are to score you high among the competitors.

The national poet of Pakistan, Dr. Muhammad Iqbal in a verse in his Urdu poetry narrates;

Tundi-e Baad-e Mukhalif se na ghabra aye ooqab

Ye to chalti hai tujhay ooncha oorhanay kay liyay

Translation:

O'eagle! not to scare of opposing, harsh wind

Thy flow fast to compel you for a higher flight

PLANNING FOR PREPARATION

P ractice is the key to success. There is a famous saying, *"Practice makes a person perfect."*

Timely practice gives you the confidence and thus results in a better performance during examination and ultimate success.

Start your preparation well before the theory exam and utilize the time between the theory and clinicals for rehearsals only.

Candidates who start rehearsal of clinicals before the declaration of theory result have brighter chances to clear the clinicals as well.

BEFORE THEORY

Perform and write down at least three long cases from all the major systems and repeat each case at least twice.

Preferably a senior and if not available even a junior colleague or alike candidate should act as your "Practice Examiner".

Try to improve the timing of History and Physical

examination; History about 15 min and Physical examination 10 min.

This quick approach will be helpfull in the short-cases as well.

During routine clinical work you can practice the components of a long-case in fractions, like sometimes History, sometimes Physicals or even a part of Physical examination, and sometimes Presentation and Discussion.

GAP BETWEEN
THEORY & CLINICALS

Perform at least two long-cases per week.

A senior colleague, better a previous examiner or at least a supervisor of PGs should act as a practice examiner at this stage. It will be useful if a pair is made with a junior colleague or alike candidate.

Take the feedback from the "Practice Examiner" after presentation; both on the content and style of presentation.

The same case should better be repeated after rectification of deficiencies pointed out by the Practice Examiner.

An example of the plan or schedule for preparation of clinicals is given below.

SCHEDULE FOR PREPARATION OF CLINICALS

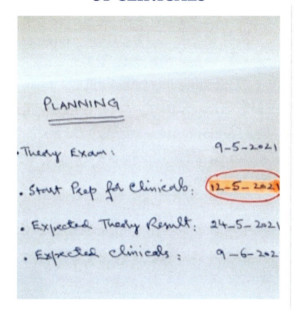

BACKGROUND KNOWLEDGE

T he original research, mostly the randomized controlled clinical trials (RCTs) which have changed the medical practice (called as land-mark trials) are always remembered and medical students, especially the postgraduate and active clinicians are expected to be familiar with these studies.

With the development of subspecialties and their societies, these trials can easily be obtained from the literature of relevant society websites.

Societies of international repute regularly publish the best clinical practice guidelines for various clinical conditions and it is mandatory for the PGs to download and save or better save the hard copies of the latest guidelines for the management of common diseases.

Some of the land-mark trials of interest with abbreviated summaries are given at the end of each chapter.

References and electronic links of important guidelines and studies are provided where appropriate.

COMMON LONG CASES

I nternal Medicine is the subject, vast like an ocean. You may come across any common or even a rare case during your exam. However, common things are common and need special emphasis and preparation. Moreover, it is important to note that some rare cases are commonly shown in the exams.

While attempting the long-case, always keep in mind that these patients usually have a disease with involvement of multiple organ systems like DM, HT, SLE.

Some of the common long-cases are listed below to be prepared and mastered as a home-work before attempting the exam. Diseases highlighted are more common and need special emphasis.

In the forthcoming section, we will discuss some of these long-cases in detail with their presentation and possible questions asked during the discussion, with material and tips to prepare for the proper answers, and the tactics to come out of the difficult situations.

LIST OF COMMON LONG-CASES

System	Cases	System	Cases
Respiratory	COPD Pleural effusion Idiopathic pulmonary fibrosis Bronchogenic carcinoma Pneumonia	Rheumatology	Rheumatoid arthritis SLE Systemic sclerosis
Cardiovascular	HT CHD Heart failure Valvular heart disease Infective endocarditis	Endocrinology	DM with complications Thyroid disease
Abdominal	CLD CKD Renal transplant Chronic diarrhea	Miscellaneous	Obesity Depression Prolonged fever HIV/AIDS Psoriasis
Neurology	Stroke Multiple sclerosis		

DIABETES MELLITUS

Diabetes mellitus is the most common long-case shown in the clinical examinations and quite a common case in the clinical practice as well. It is truly said *"if you know the diabetes, you know the Medicine and vice versa"*.

Diabetes is a multisystem disorder and patients can present with a wide range of complications. Moreover, diabetic patients usually have HT as well and this makes them a suitable case for discussion.

The summary and management plan of a typical patient with both diabetes and HT is given below.

SUMMARY

This gentleman, Mr. Malik, 58 years old, from D.I.Khan city, is suffering from type 2 diabetes and HT for the last 12 years. Currently he presented with burning sensation of both his feet for the last two months.

On examination; his pulse rate is 74 beats/min, regular, BP sitting 170/105 mmHg, standing 165/102 mmHg (on medications - Amlodipine + Valsartan 5/160).

Examination of chest, heart, and abdomen is unremarkable.

CNS examination revealed diminished vibration sense distally in both the lower limbs and fundoscopy showed widespread hard exudates and micro-aneurysms sparing the macular region.

He has got:

Type 2 diabetes with peripheral neuropathy + background diabetic retinopathy, and HT which is not well-controlled.

MANAGEMENT PLAN

After assessing the diabetic status by performing the post-prandial & fasting blood sugar and HbA1c, I will adjust his anti-diabetic medications and aim at the tight glycemic control i.e. FBS <130 mg/dl, RBS <160 mg/dl, and HbA1c <7% - Targets of treatment according to the American Diabetic Association (ADA).

I will also check some basic investigations like FBC, U&Es, and MSU with microscopy.

I will check his urinary micro-albumin - an early sign of nephropathy and his lipid profile.

For better control of HT, I would like to increase the dose of his current medications (CCB+ARB), and add a thiazide diuretic to aim at the good BP control i.e. <140/90 mmHg (Target of treatment according to the JNC-8).

For control of diabetes, I would like to adjust his doses as recommended by the ADA guidelines.

For peripheral neuropathy, I will prescribe symptomatic treatment like gabalin or pregabalin and vitamin B12 supplements.

As he doesn't have any acute complication of DM or HT

at the moment, he doesn't need hospitalization and can be managed at home with planned follow-ups.

For retinopathy I will refer the patient to an ophthalmologist for proper assessment and necessary treatment if required, apart from the tight glycemic control.

I will identify and manage the risk factors like smoking, hypercholesterolemia and arrange for patient's education and counseling.

I will address his social, occupational, and dietary needs including lifestyle changes, exercise, and will arrange for a medic-alert identification bracelet.

I will suggest his GP to assess the response to treatment by regular monitoring of his diabetic status (FBS, RBS, HbA1c) and BP.

DISCUSSION

During discussion, most of the questions will revolve around the diagnosis, management and complications of DM &/or HT.

Some tips are given below to help organize your answers.

DIABETES MELLITUS

Diabetes is a disorder of carbohydrates, lipids, and proteins metabolism characterized by hyperglycemia due to insufficient or inefficient insulin that results in a wide range of complications.

It has two main types.

- Type 1 diabetes
- Type 2 diabetes

Apart from these two major types there are some other variants like:

Gestational diabetes: Diabetes that develops or is first recognized during pregnancy.

Secondary diabetes: Like post-pancreatitis, panceatectomy, hormonal disorders like Cushing's syndrome, certain drugs like corticosteroids.

Other specific types: Certain genetic variants.

DIAGNOSTIC CRITERIA

According to the WHO:

- FBS ≥126 mg/dl (7 mmol/l).
- 2-Hr postprandial ≥200 mg/dl (11.1 mmol/l).

If one of these is abnormal, the other should be performed on another day.

GTT should be performed in individuals with FBS 110-125 mg/dl (6.1–6.9 mmol/l) to determine the glucose tolerance status.

GLUCOSE
TOLERANCE TEST

It measures the body's ability to metabolize glucose.

Patient reports to the lab in a fasting state and blood and urine samples for sugar are collected. Then he is given 75 G glucose orally.

In modified GTT, samples for blood and urine sugar are taken at 1-Hr and 2-Hr post-glucose.

GLUCOSE TOLERANCE TEST

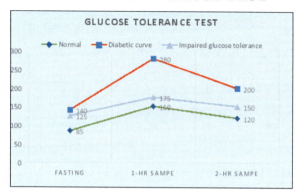

Figure 2.1: Typical curves of glucose tolerance test in normal, diabetic, and impaired tolerance.

INTERPRETATION OF PLASMA GLUCOSE VALUES

Glucose status	Fasting mmol/l (mg/dl)	1-h post-glucose mmol/l (mg/dl)	2-h post-glucose mmol/l (mg/dl)
Normal	<7.0 (126)	<11.1 (200)	< 7.8 (<140)
Diabetes	>7.0 (>126)	>11.1 (200)	> 11.1 (>200)
Impaired glucose tolerance	<7.0 (<126)	<11.1 (200)	7.8–11.0 (140–199)
Impaired fasting glucose	5.6-6.9 (100–125)	-	-

MANAGEMENT

Doctor-patient relationship and patient education has a pivotal role in the management of diabetes.

The goals of treatment are to alleviate the symptoms and prevent the complications.

Both non-pharmacologic and pharmacologic measures are equally important.

Dietary restrictions and regular exercise are the most important non-pharmacologic measures.

Measures to avoid the CV risk factors like cessation of smoking, moderation of alcohol intake, and weight reduction also has immense importance in the management.

GOAL: DIABETIC CONTROL OR CURE

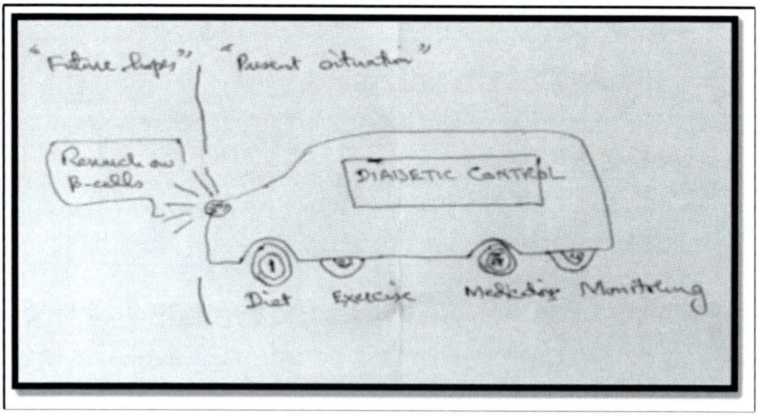

Figure 2.2: Food for thought: artistic presentation of the present situation and future hopes.

DRUGS USED IN DIABETES

Insulin:

It is the only choice of therapy for type 1 diabetes, gestational diabetes, and during severe illness. However, for the rest of the patients it is also the first choice of therapy with other options as well.

Insulin has many types depending upon its onset and duration of action.

Proper scheduling of the type according to the need or situation helps in the proper glycemic control.

Oral anti-diabetics:

- Sulphonyl ureas
- Biguanides
- Thiazolidines (Glitazones)
- Alpha-glucosidase inhibitors
- DPP-4 inhibitors (Gliptins)
- Meglitinides (Glinides)
- Amylin analogues
- GLP-1 and GLP-2 analogues

Any class of the anti-diabetic drugs can be discussed with special emphasis on its beneficial edge over the others and its side-effects.

TYPES OF INSULIN AND THEIR PHARMACOKINETICS

Type	Onset (hours)	Peak (hours)	Duration (hours)
Aspart Glulisine Lispro	0.2-0.5	0.5-2	3-4
Regular	0.5-1	2-3	6-8
NPH	1.5	4-10	16-24
Lente	1.5-3	7-15	16-24
Ultra-lente	3-4	9-15	22-28
Glargine Detemir	1-2	-	24-36 18-24

COMPLICATIONS

Acute:
- DKA
- Hypoglycemia
- Hyperosmolar state
- Lactic acidosis

Chronic:
- **Microvascular:**

Neuropathy
Nephropathy
Retinopathy
- **Macrovascular:**

Cerebrovascular disease
Coronary heart disease
Peripheral vascular disease
- **Other:**

Diabetic foot
Diabetic dermopathy
Cataract

You must be clear and well-versed regarding the pathology and management of all these complications. Any of these can be discussed in details. Some of these complications are discussed in the pages to follow.

DIABETIC RETINOPATHY

Background: Hard exudates and micro-aneurysms.

Pre-proliferative: Soft exudates and flame-shaped hemorrhages.

Proliferative: Neovascularization.

Advanced: Proliferative retinopathy with complications like fibrosis or vitreous hemorrhage.

DIABETIC KETOACIDOSIS

D iabetic ketoacidosis (DKA) is the most serious complication of diabetes. It mostly occurs in type-1 diabetics. It is characterized by:

- Hyperglycaemia: >250 mg/dl
- Acidosis: Arterial blood pH <7.3
- Low serum bicarbonate: <15 mEq/l
- Serum ketones: Positive

INVESTIGATIONS

- Blood glucose, Plasma ketones, ABGs, U&Es
- FBC, Urinalysis, ECG, Chest x-ray
- Blood & urine cultures, S. amylase, Cardiac enzymes

MANAGEMENT

- **IV line:** Two wide-bore cannulae - one for fluids, and other for insulin.
- **Fluid replacement:** With normal renal function - 4L over first 4 hours.

[Normal saline 1L IVI over 15 min, then 1L over 30 min, 1L over 1 hour, and 1L over next 2 hours].

Then Normal saline 1L 6 hourly.

Switch to 5% Dextrose when blood sugar <300 mg/dl.

- **Insulin:** Estimate blood glucose hourly.

Soluble insulin 10 units IV STAT. Then 4-8 units/hr IV infusion.

Decrease to 2-4 U/hr when blood sugar <250 mg/dl.

Switch to "Physiologic SC scale" when fully conscious, can take orally and ketones are cleared.

- **Potassium:** Serum K$^+$ estimated every 2 hrs.

Caution: Potassium is always given by slow IV infusion; rapid infusion may lead to cardiac arrest.

3.5-5.5 mmol /l	20 mmol /l
<3.5 mmol /l	40 mmol /l
>5.5 mmol /l	Nil

- **NG tube:** Required for suction; if the patient has nausea /vomiting.
- **Treat the precipitants:** Infection: Parenteral antibiotics (third generation cephalosporin)
- **Be alert to complications:**

  Shock: Inotropes

  Cerebral edema: 20% Mannitol 200 ml IVI rapid over 15 min

  DIC: FFP

  DVT: Heparin 5,000 units SC BD.

HYPOGLYCEMIA

Hypoglycemia is not uncommon during the course of treatment of DM. Tight glycemic control is desired at the cost of occasional hypoglycemia. Patients must be educated to avoid hypoglycemia by adjusting the dosage of their anti-diabetic agents and timings of food intake.

Symptoms of hypoglycemia are hunger, sweating, sinking of heart, palpitation, tremulousness, confusion, and coma.

In the emergency situation when a patient is suspected to have hypoglycemia on clinical grounds: Check the blood glucose if feasible without wasting the time.

MANAGEMENT

- **If the patient is alert:**

Oral glucose: Like fruit Juice followed by carbohydrate-rich diet.

- **If the patient is drowsy or in coma:**

50 ml of 50% glucose IV. (Preceded by Thiamin 100 mg IV).

Repeat the same if required.

Then 10% glucose 1L IVI BD.

- **If on insulin:**

Once stable; adjust the dose and send him home with counseling to avoid the situation in future.

· **If on oral anti-diabetics:**

Admit. Continue monitoring and 10% glucose 1L IVI BD for 48 hours.

Note: There are 101 causes of hypoglycemia, diabetes is only one of these, consider other causes of hypoglycemia as well.

HYPEROSMOLAR HYPERGLYCEMIC STATE

Characteristic features:

- Hyperglycaemia: >600 mg/dl
- Serum osmolality: >310 mOsm/kg
- No acidosis: Arterial blood pH >7.3
- Serum bicarbonate >15 mEq/l
- Normal anion gap: <14 mEq/l

MANAGEMENT
- Fluid replacement
- Insulin (Smaller doses as compared to DKA)
- Potassium
- Phosphates

LACTIC ACIDOSIS

Characteristic features:

- Severe acidosis with hyperventilation: pH <7.3
- Low serum bicarbonate: <15 mEq/l
- High anion gap: >15 mEq/l
- Serum ketones: Negative
- Serum lactate: >5 mmol/l

PREDISPOSING FACTORS

- Metformin therapy
- Renal impairment
- Tissue hypoxia
- Liver failure

MANAGEMENT

- Treatment of predisposing cause.

- Adequate oxygenation.

- Vascular perfusion of tissues.

- Alkalinization: Sodium bicarbonate infusion to keep the arterial pH >7.5 (Up-to 2000 mEq in 24 hours).

- Hemodialysis: In more severe cases.

SUBCUTANEOUS SLIDING-SCALE INSULIN

Historically subcutaneous sliding-scale insulin was prescribed for diabetic patients admitted to the hospital. Despite lot of controversy regarding its metabolic benefits it remained in common practice for a long time.

Although now obsolete but it is given below for the intrested readers.

Check blood glucose and give insulin accordingly:
Before breakfast
Before lunch
Before dinner
At bed-time

If NPO, check glucose and give regular insulin 4 hourly.

SUBCUTANEOUS SLIDING-SCALE INSULIN

Blood glucose (mg/dl)	Soluble insulin (Units)
40 or below	Nil (Give 50 ml of 50% glucose)
41-75	Nil
76-125	2
126-200	4
201-300	6
301-400	8
> 400	10 (Call the Doctor)

PHYSIOLOGIC SC INSULIN PROTOCOL

It is a physiologically better alternative to the traditional "SC sliding-scale insulin". Insulin is given as three dosage schedule:

- **Basal insulin:** The initial total daily dose of insulin is calculated using a factor of 0.3 to 0.6 Units/kg body weight, and half of it is given as long-acting insulin.
- **Nutritional insulin:** The other half is divided over three meals as short-acting insulin.
- **Correctional insulin:** Based on the pre-prandial blood glucose results, it provides the final insulin adjustment.

Studies have demonstrated reduction in hyperglycemic measurements, hypoglycemia, and adjusted hospital length of stay with physiologic SC insulin protocols.

LAND-MARK TRIALS

· UKPDS
United Kingdom Prospective Diabetes Study

> This study established the importance of tight glycemic control in reducing the risk and progress of microvascular complications.

In this study, 5102 patients with newly diagnosed type 2 DM were randomized to intensive therapy, which achieved a median HbA1c of 7% compared with conventional therapy with a median HbA1c 7.9% and followed for 10 years.

In addition, 1148 patients who were also hypertensive were randomized to "tight" BP control (goal BP<150/85 mmHg) or "less tight" (goal BP<180/105 mmHg).

Microvascular complications i.e. retinopathy, nephropathy, and possibly neuropathy were benefited while macrovascular complications were not significantly lowered by tight glycemic control.

Tight control of BP in type 2 DM reduced the risk of both micro and macrovascular complications (MI, sudden death, stroke, PVD), along with diabetes-related mortality.

Ref: Br J Clin Pharmacol 999; 48:643–8.

. DCCT
Diabetes Control and Complications Trial

In insulin dependent DM intensive therapy effectively delays the onset and slows the progression of diabetic retinopathy, nephropathy, and neuropathy.

In this study, 1441 patients with type 1 DM were randomized to two groups; one treated convention-ally (goal: clinical well-being; called standard treatment group) and another treated intensively (goal: normal-ization of blood glucose; called intensive treatment group) and followed for 7 years.

Intensive treatment group was clearly distinguished from standard treatment group in terms of glycated hemoglobin and blood glucose values. There was sig-nificant reduction in the risk of diabetic retinopathy, nephropathy, and neuropathy in intensive treatment group. The benefit of intensive therapy resulted in delay in the onset and slowing of progression of these compli-cations.

Ref: N Engl J Med 1993; 329:977-86.

. FDPS
Finish Diabetes Prevention Study

This study showed the significance of intensive life-style intervention (Diet-exercise program) producing long-term beneficial changes leading to reduced risk of type 2 DM.

In this study, 523 overweight subjects with IGT were randomized to either intervention or control group. The main measure in intervention group was individual dietary advice aimed at reducing weight and intake of saturated fats and increasing dietary fibre. They were individually guided to increase their level of physical activity, while control group received general information about the benefits of weight reduction, physical activity and healthy diet in prevention of DM.

Pilot study began in 1993, and recruitment ended in 1998. By 1999 there were 65 new cases of DM, 34 dropouts and one death. Weight reduction was greater at 1 year in intervention than control group and this difference was sustained in the second year of follow-up. At 1 year the intervention group showed significantly greater reductions in 2h glucose, fasting and 2h insulin, systolic and diastolic BP, and triglycerides. Most of the beneficial changes in CV risk factors were sustained for 2 years.

Ref: Br J Nutr 2000; 83 Suppl 1:S137-42.

· DPP
Diabetes Prevention Program

This study provided a detailed description of the highly successful lifestyle intervention for prevention of DM.

In this study, 1079 participants which included 45% racial and ethnic minorities were subjected to lifestyle intervention with the goal of minimum 7% weight loss/maintenance and a minimum of 150 min physical activity similar in intensity to brisk walk. Methods used to achieve these lifestyle goals included:

1) individual case managers or lifestyle coaches;

2) frequent contact with participants;

3) a structured, state-of-the-art, 16-session core curriculum that taught behavioral self-management strategies for weight loss and physical activity;

4) supervised physical activity sessions;

5) a more flexible maintenance intervention, combining group and individual approaches, motivational campaigns, and restarts;

6) individualization through a toolbox of adherence strategies;

7) tailoring of materials and strategies to address ethnic diversity; and

8) an extensive network of training, feedback, and clinical support.

Lifestyle intervention resulted in 58% reduction in the incidence of DM.

Ref: Diabetes Care 2002; 25: 2165-71.

HYPERTENSION

Hypertension can present in a variety of patterns and the patients can be discussed in various modules as follows:

- **Essential HT:**

Mild to Moderate HT without any complication.
Moderate to severe HT associated with target-organ damage.
Severe HT with acute complication.

- **Secondary HT:**

RAS
Cushing's syndrome
Coarctation of aorta
Conn's syndrome
Pheochromocytoma
PIH

- **HT associated with:**

DM, IHD, Obesity, Dyslipidemia, renal disease.

Patient-1: **SUMMARY**

This gentleman, Mr. Gandapur, 60 years old, from Kulachi, is having HT for the last 20 years. He presented this time with weakness of right half of the body and motor dysphasia a day earlier, which recovered completely.

On examination; his pulse is 68 bpm, and BP 200/110 mmHg (on medications CCB+ARB). Examination of chest, heart, and abdomen is unremarkable.

CNS examination didn't reveal any focal neurological deficit at the moment.

Fundoscopy showed grade-2 hypertensive changes i.e. arteriolar thickening and AV nipping.

He has got:

HT with TIA and grade 2 hypertensive retinopathy

MANAGEMENT PLAN

I will perform some basic investigations like FBC, U&Es, and MSU and investigations as guided by the given scenario of H&P with the aim:

To determine the cause and risk factors like lipid profile. To determine the complications like RFTs and to determine the associated conditions like blood sugar.

For better control of HT, I would like to increase the dose of his current medications (CCB+ARB) and add a thiazide diuretic to aim at the BP <140/90 mmHg - Target of treatment according to the Joint National Committee on prevention, detection, evaluation, and treatment, of high BP (JNC)-8.

As he is having hypertensive urgency at the moment, he needs hospitalization and to bring the BP gradually down to a reasonable level (can be discussed by the examiner as given in the discussion section).

I will identify and stratify the risk factors for heart like smoking, hypercholesterolemia and arrange for patient's education and counseling.

I will address his social, occupational, and dietary needs including the lifestyle changes and exercise.

I will suggest his GP to assess the response to treatment by regular monitoring of his condition including the BP.

Patient-2:

SUMMARY

This gentleman, Mr. Patail, 35 years age, a business-man by profession from Lahore, presented with irrit-ability, and pain in the back of his neck and occiput for few days. It is pulsatile in character, mostly present in the day-time and is relieved at night while asleep. At times he also feels dizzy. There is no history of fever. His mother had HT and died of stroke.

On examination; he is a normal built gentleman (BMI 26 kg/m^2). Pulse rate is 72 bpm, regular with no radio-femoral delay and BP is 220/110 mmHg (on Atenolol 50 mg daily).

Heart examination revealed a heaving apex beat in the 5th intercostal space at the mid clavicular line. Heart sounds are normal with no added sound. Examination of the chest, and abdomen is unremarkable.

CNS examination didn't reveal any focal neurological deficit. There is no neck rigidity or Kernig's sign. Fundoscopy showed grade III hypertensive changes i.e. soft exudates and flame-shaped hemorrhages.

My provisional diagnosis is:

Severe HT with probable hypertensive encephalop-athy and evidence of target-organ damage i.e. ret-inopathy.

MANAGEMENT PLAN

I will perform some basic investigations like FBC, U&Es, blood sugar, and MSU and investigations pertaining to my provisional diagnosis like CT scan or MRI of brain, RFTs, to establish the diagnosis.

As he is having hypertensive emergency, he needs hospitalization and to bring the BP gradually down to a reasonable level (can be discussed by the examiner as given in the discussion section).

Once stable, I will identify and stratify the risk factors for heart like smoking, hypercholesterolemia and arrange for patient's education and counseling.

I will address his social, occupational, and dietary needs including the lifestyle changes and exercise.

On discharge, I would suggest his GP to assess the response to treatment by regular monitoring of his condition including the BP.

Patient-3:

SUMMARY

This lady Mrs. Begum 46 years old who had been hypertensive for the last 6 years on tablet hydromet (methyl dopa + hydrochlorothiazide). Initially she was tried on ACE-I and ARB to which she was found resistant. On one summer while coming back from the market, she felt profound weakness in her lower limbs. She also noticed that she could not get up from sitting position during prayers. On system review she revealed loose motions for few days.

On examination she has bilateral, symmetrical partial ptosis with normal eye-ball movements. Her pulse is 78 bpm, BP 160/110 mmHg in lying position in the right arm.

Neurological examination is normal except bilateral mild ptosis with normal ocular movements and proximal muscle weakness. Heart examination revealed heaving apex beat in the 5th intercostal space at the mid clavicular line. CNS examination didn't reveal any focal neurological deficit. Chest, heart, and abdominal examination are unremarkable.

Fundoscopy showed grade III hypertensive changes i.e. soft exudates and flame-shaped hemorrhages.

My provisional diagnosis is:

Secondary HT probably due to Conn's syndrome

MANAGEMENT PLAN

I will perform some basic investigations like FBC, U&Es, and MSU and investigations as guided by the given scenario of H&P with the aim to determine the cause, complications and risk factors like: USG of abdomen, CT/MRI abdomen, plasma aldosterone level.

As he is having hypertensive emergency, he needs hospitalization and to bring the BP gradually down to a reasonable level (can be discussed by the examiner as given in the discussion section).

Once stable, I will identify and stratify the risk factors for heart like smoking, hypercholesterolemia and arrange for patient's education and counseling.

I will address his social, occupational, and dietary needs including the lifestyle changes and exercise.

On discharge, I would suggest his GP to assess the response to treatment by regular monitoring of his condition including the BP.

Patient-4:

SUMMARY

This gentleman, Mr. Zeeshan, 35 years age, a businessman by profession from Lahore, presented with irritability, and pain in the upper neck and occiput. At times he feels dizzy. This 50 years old lady who had been hypertensive for the last 5 years on tablets. She felt profound weakness in her lower limbs.

On examination her pulse was 74 bpm, BP 165/115 mmHg. He has a bruite on right renal area.

Chest and heart examination was unremarkable.

CNS examination didn't reveal any focal neurological deficit.

Fundoscopy showed grade II hypertensive changes.

My provisional diagnosis is:

Secondary HT probably due to RAS

MANAGEMENT PLAN

I will perform some basic investigations like FBC, U&Es, and MSU and investigations as guided by the given scenario of H&P with the aim to determine the cause lie USG of abdomen, CT abdomen, renal angiography, plasma aldosterone level.

He needs hospitalization and to bring the BP gradually down to a reasonable level (can be discussed by the examiner as given in the discussion section).

Once stable and confirmed I will refer her to the proper specialty for definitive treatment like renal angioplasty.

I will identify and stratify the risk factors for heart like smoking, hypercholesterolemia and arrange for patient's education and counseling.

I will address his social, occupational, and dietary needs including the lifestyle changes and exercise.

On discharge, I would suggest his GP to assess the response to treatment by regular monitoring of his condition including the BP.

HISTORY

Age: If young; consider secondary HT like coarctation of aorta.

Gender: In ladies consider PIH.

Presenting complaints: Mild to moderate HT can be discovered incidentally on routine medical check-up.

Symptoms suggestive of severe HT: Like headache, palpitations, nausea /vomiting, SOB.

Symptoms related to target-organ damage:

CNS: TIA, stroke, hypertensive encephalopathy.

CVS: Palpitations (arrhythmias), angina, SOB (heart failure).

Renal: Nausea/vomiting, pallor, puffiness of face (CRF).

Symptoms related to associated condition: DM, hyper/hypothyroidism, IHD, obesity, arteriosclerosis (palpable vessel wall, xanthelasma).

Systemic review for target-organ damage: Blurring of vision, muscles weakness, speech problem, dizziness, LOC, puffiness of face, swelling of feet, urinary problem.

Family history: Family history of obesity, HT, DM, dyslipidemia may be present in essential HT. APKD is an autosomal dominant condition.

CLINICAL EXAMINATION

GPE

Facies: Pale, sallow in CRF, plethoric face in Cushing's syndrome, polycythemia.

Body habitus: Obesity in metabolic syndrome.

Pulse: If bradycardia, consider hypothyroidism, β-blockers. Tachycardia, consider thyrotoxicosis. Fixed rate heart-beat, consider dysautonomia due to DM.

Irregular pulse can be due to AF or multiple ectopics. Ignore the variation in intensity of beats and note the faintest of Korotkoff sounds.

In paroxysmal HT consider pheochromocytoma.

Identify HT by clinic BP and confirm by home readings or ABPM:

Method of checking BP: The rule of two: Sitting /standing; Palpatory /auscultatory method; twice on one occasion; cuff 2 fingers above the cubital fossa; palpate the two arteries (radial and brachial).

Grade the HT: Like in NICE guidelines.

Look for possible cause:

Radio-femoral delay - coarctation of aorta (if so check BP in the legs).

Renal artery bruite - RAS.

Palpable kidneys - APKD.

Look for target-organ damage:

Heart: Arrhythmias, Cardiomegaly, Hepatomegaly.

Fundi: Hypertensive retinopathy. Athersclerotic changes may be associated with or the effect of HT. Associated diabetic changes may also be present.

Renal: Early impairment or late stage with all signs of ESRD.

Neurology: Muscles weakness (↓ K) /hemiparesis.

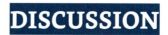

DISCUSSION

HYPERTENSION

P ersistent elevation of BP to a level at which the treatment would be beneficial for the patient is called hypertension (HT). According to the "Joint National Committee for detection, treatment and prevention of hypertension" (JNC)-8, BP $\geq$140/90 mmHg is labelled as HT.

High systolic ($\geq$160 mmHg) with normal diastolic BP is labelled as "Isolated systolic HT" (ISH).

HT is the most common cardiovascular disease with a global prevalence of 10-20%.

GRADING
According to the NICE clinical guidelines.

Stage 1: Clinic BP $\geq$140/90 mmHg and subsequent ABPM average $\geq$135/95 mmHg.

Stage 2: Clinic BP $\geq$160/100 mmHg and subsequent ABPM average $\geq$150/95 mmHg.

Severe: Clinic SBP $\geq$180 mmHg or DBP $\geq$110 mmHg.

White coat effect:
A discrepancy of 20/10 mmHg between the clinic BP and average day-time ABPM or average home BP monitoring.

INVESTIGATIONS

According to the NICE guidelines the purpose of investigations is:

- To search for the cause.
- To assess the target-organ damage and cardiovascular
  risk.

Those with young age, severe HT, and no family history are thoroughly investigated to rule out any secondary cause.

U&Es, Blood sugar, Urinalysis & microscopy

Chest x-ray, ECG

Creatinine

Lipid profile

Calcium

Renal USG, IVU, renal angiography

Urinary VMA, urinary free cortisol

EVIDENCE OF TARGET-ORGAN DAMAGE

Heart: Cardiac enlargement, ECG showing LVH with strain pattern. Angina, MI, LVF, CCF.

Kidneys: Proteinuria, Impaired renal function, ESRD

Brain: TIA, Stroke.

Eyes: Keith-Wagener-Barker classification:

Grade I: Arteriolar thickening, silver wiring.

Grade II: AV nipping.

Grade III: Cotton-wool (soft) exudates and flame-shaped hemorrhages, macular edema.

Grade IV: Papilledema.

CAUSES

Primary or essential   95%

Secondary   5%

CAUSES OF
SECONDARY HYPERTENSION

Renal causes:

- Acute and Chronic Glomerulonephritis
- Chronic pyelonephritis
- Renal A stenosis
- Polycystic kidney disease
- Connective tissue disorders: Polyarteritis nodosa, Systemic sclerosis
- Diabetic nephropathy

Endocrine causes:

- Pheochromocytoma
- Cushing's syndrome
- Conn's syndrome (Pri. hyperaldosteronism)
- Congenital adrenal hyperplasia
- Other: Acromegaly, Hyperparathyroidism, Hypo and hyperthyroidism

Cardiovascular causes:

Coarctation of aorta

Other causes:

- Pre-eclampsia /eclampsia
- Drugs: NSAIDs, corticosteroids, estrogen-containing OCPs, anabolic steroids, sympathomimetic agents, EPO.
- Alcohol

RISK FACTORS

Non-modifiable:

- **Age:** BP rises with increasing age, in both the genders.
- **Genetic factors:** Children of hypertensive parents have 45% possibility of developing HT, as compared to 3% with normotensive parents. First degree relatives show significantly increased values.

Modifiable:

- Obesity
- High salt intake
- High saturated fat intake
- Alcohol
- Physical inactivity
- Environmental stress
- Secondary causes

MANAGEMENT

Non-Pharmacologic:
- Optimize the weight
- Regular exercise
- Healthy diet
- Avoid table salt
- Stop smoking
- Reduce alcohol intake to $\leq$ 1 unit/day
- Relaxation therapy

Pharmacologic:
- Thiazide diuretics
- Beta blockers
- Calcium channel blockers
- ACE-Inhibitors /ARBs
- Vasodilators
- Centrally acting drugs

ADVERSE EFFECTS OF ANTI-HYPERTENSIVE DRUGS

Thiazide diuretics: Hypokalemia, hyperuricemia.

Calcium channel blockers: Pedal edema, Constipation, reflex tachycardia.

Beta blockers: Bronchospasm, heart block, hypercholesterolemia.

ACE-inhibitors /ARBs: Cough (common with ACE-I), postural hypotension, angio-edema.

PROGNOSIS

HT is the 2nd most common cause of death in developed countries. Higher the BP, greater the risk of mortality and reduction in life expectancy. Death is mainly due to its complications: Heart disease (CAD, heart failure), stroke, and renal failure.

Bad prognostic signs:

- Male sex, young age, black race
- Severe HT
- Smoking
- DM
- Hypercholesterolemia
- Obesity
- Evidence of target-organ damage

PREVENTION

WHO recommendations:

- Reduce the salt intake (to less than 5g daily).
- Eat more fruit and vegetables.
- Be physically active on a regular basis.
- Avoid the use of tobacco.
- Reduce alcohol consumption.
- Limit the intake of foods high in saturated fats.
- Eliminate /reduce trans fats in the diet.

HYPERTENSIVE EMERGENCIES

V ery high BP (Systolic >180 or diastolic >120 mmgh) can lead to acute target-organ damage.

Hypertensive urgency: Very high BP without acute target-organ damage.

Hypertensive emergency: Very high BP with acute target-organ damage.

Hypertensive emergency may present as:
- Hypertensive encephalopathy
- Acute LVF
- Aortic dissection
- Acute coronary syndrome
- Intracranial hemorrhage
- Acute renal failure

DRUGS USED IN HYPERTENSIVE EMERGENCY

Following parenteral drugs are commonly used to quickly lower the BP.

Once adequate BP level is obtained, oral drugs are started and parenteral gradually weaned off.

The choice of drug depends upon the specific organ at risk.

SODIUM NITROPRUSSIDE

A short-acting agent; the BP response is titrated from minute to minute - monitored in ICU.

It decreases systemic vascular resistance by causing direct dilatation of arterioles and veins.

It may cause intracerebral shunting, thereby increasing the ICP and should be avoided in patients suspected of having increased ICP.

Thiocyanate and cyanide toxicity can occur with prolonged use or if the patient has renal or hepatic failure.

LABETALOL

Both α and β blocker. It is particularly preferred in patients with aortic dissection and ESRD.

Because of nonselective β-blocking properties, it should be avoided in severe reactive airway disease and cardiogenic shock.

Can be given in boluses of 10-20 mg or infused at 1 mg/min until the desired BP is obtained.

ESMOLOL

It is ultra short-acting, selective β-1 receptor blocker but has little or no effect on β-2 receptors.

It is particularly useful in patients, if surgery is planned. It has been shown to reduce episodes of chest pain and clinical cardiac events.

It is useful in patients at risk for experiencing complications from β-blockade, particularly those with reactive airway disease, mild-to-moderate LV dysfunction, or peripheral vascular disease.

Its short half-life (8 minutes) allows easy titration to

the desired effect and quick discontinuance if necessary.

NICARDIPINE

It is second-generation dihydropyridine-derivative CCB, with high vascular selectivity and strong cerebral and coronary vasodilatory activity.

It increases the stroke volume and coronary blood flow. It has a potent and rapid onset of action, is easy to titrate, and lacks toxic metabolites.

PHENTOLAMINE

It is α-1 and α-2 adrenergic blocking agent that blocks the action of circulating epinephrine and norepinephrine, reducing the BP that results from catecholamine effects on the α-receptors.

HYDRALAZINE

Hydralazine is a direct arteriolar dilator. It can cause reflex tachycardia resulting in increased cardiac oxygen demand. Should be avoided in patients suspected of having increased ICP.

NITROGLYCERIN

It provides arteriolar dilation and venodilation. It is used in emergencies involving myocardial ischemia because of its dilatory effects on the coronary arteries.

HYPERTENSIVE ENCEPHALOPATHY

V ery high BP ($\geq$180/120 mmHg) with papilledema, disordered consciousness or fits. Focal neurologic deficits are infrequent

The acute rise in BP exceeds the cerebral autoregulatory range, resulting in hydrostatic leakage across the capillaries within the CNS. Persistent elevation of BP leads to arteriolar damage and necrosis leading to generalized vasodilatation, cerebral edema, and papilledema.

MRI scans have shown a pattern of typically posterior (occipital > frontal) brain edema, termed as posterior reversible encephalopathy syndrome (PRES).

MANAGEMENT

According to the American College of Cardiology/ American Heart Association (ACC/AHA) 2017 guidelines:

Admit the patient to ICU for continuous BP monitoring, monitoring for target organ damage, and for parenteral administration of appropriate medication.

Labetalol, Nicardipine, or Esmolol are the preferred medications.

Nitroprusside and hydralazine should be avoided as these agents pose a theoretical risk of intracranial shunting of blood and should be avoided in patients suspected of having increased ICP.

When therapy is initiated, it is important to consider the baseline BP to avoid excessive BP reduction and prevent cerebral ischemia.

It is usually safe to reduce the MAP by 25% and to lower the DBP to 100-110 mmHg.

Also watch for the adverse effects or toxicity of drug given.

If the neurologic deterioration worsens with therapy, it is necessary to reconsider the extent of BP reduction or to consider alternate diagnoses.

LAND-MARK TRIALS

. VA Cooperative Study I
Veterans Administration Cooperative Study I

This study established the benefits of treating severe diastolic HT.

In this RCT, 143 men with DBP 115–129 mmHg were randomized to HCT, reserpine, hydralazine added in a step-wise fashion or placebo.

The trial was stopped early at 18 months because 27 severe complications and 4 deaths occurred in placebo group as compared to 2 severe complications and 0 deaths in active group.

Ref: JAMA 1967; 202:1028-34.

. VA Cooperative Study II

In patients with mild to moderate HT, lowering DBP preserves the target organs.

In this RCT, 380 hypertensive men with DBP 90–114 mmHg were randomized to HCT, reserpine, hydralazine added in step-wise fashion or placebo and followed for 5 years.

Placebo group had higher morbidity from heart failure, stroke, and renal failure and deaths as compared to treatment group.

Ref: JAMA 1970; 213:1143-52.

· HDFP

Hypertension, Detection, and Follow-up Program

> This study established the efficacy of treating adults with mild diastolic HT, irrespective of race or gender.

In this community-based, RCT involving 10,940 persons with high BP, comparing the effects on five-year mortality of a systematic antihypertensive treatment program (Stepped Care [SC]) and referral to community medical therapy (Referred Care [RC]). Participants, recruited by population-based screening of 158,906 people aged 30-69 years in 14 communities throughout the US, were randomly assigned to SC or RC groups within each center and by entry DBP (90-104, 105 to 114, and 115+ mmHg).

Over the five years of study, more than two third SC participants continued to receive medication, and >50% achieved BP levels within the normotensive range. Control of BP was consistently better for SC than RC group. Five-year mortality from all causes was 17% lower for SC compared to RC group (P<0.01) and 20% lower for SC subgroup with entry DBP 90 to 104 mmHg compared to the corresponding RC subgroup (P<0.01).

Ref: JAMA 1979; 242:2562-71.

. SHEP
Systolic Hypertension in the Elderly Program

> Treating isolated systolic HT in older patients with diuretics reduces the stroke and cardiac endpoints.

In this RCT, 4736 men and women aged $\geq$60 with isolated systolic HT at 16 clinical centers in US were randomly assigned to receive 12.5 mg/d chlorthalidone (step 1); 25 mg/d atenolol or 0.05 mg/d reserpine (step 2) could be added; or placebo with average follow-up 4.5 years.

85 & 132 participants in active treatment and placebo groups respectively had ischemic strokes (adjusted RR, 0.63; 95% CI, 0.48-0.82); 9 & 19 had hemorrhagic strokes (adjusted RR, 0.46; 95% CI, 0.21-1.02); and 9 & 8 had strokes of unknown type (adjusted RR, 1.05; 95% CI, 0.40-2.73). Four subtypes of ischemic stroke were observed in active treatment and placebo group, as follows: for lacunar, n=23 and n=43 (adjusted RR, 0.53; 95% CI, 0.32-0.88); for embolic, n=9 and n=16 (adjusted RR, 0.56; 95% CI, 0.25-1.27); for atherosclerotic, n=13 and n=13 (adjusted RR, 0.99; 95% CI, 0.46-2.15); and for unknown subtype, n=40 and n=60 (adjusted RR, 0.64; 95% CI, 0.43-0.96). Treatment effect was observed within 1 year for hemorrhagic but not seen until 2nd year for ischemic strokes. Stroke incidence significantly decreased in participants attaining study-specific systolic BP goals.

Ref: JAMA 2000; 284:465-71.

. SYS-EUR
The European Working Party on High BP in Elderly

> Treating isolated systolic HT in elderly patients with CCB reduces the stroke and cardiac endpoints.

All patients (>60 years) were initially started on masked placebo. At three run-in visits 1 month apart, their average sitting SBP was 160-219 mmHg with DBP <95 mmHg. After stratification for centre, sex, and previous CV complications, 4695 patients were randomly assigned to nitrendipine 10-40 mg daily, with the possible addition of enalapril 5-20 mg daily and HCT 12.5-25 mg daily, or matching placebos.

At median 2 years' follow-up, sitting systolic and diastolic BPs had fallen by 13 and 2 mmHg in placebo group (n=2297) and 23 and 7 in active treatment group (n=2398). The between-group differences were systolic 10.1 mmHg (95% CI 8.8-11.4) and diastolic 4.5 mmHg (3.9-5.1). Active treatment reduced the rate of stroke from 13.7 to 7.9 endpoints per 1000 patient-years (42% reduction; p=0.003). Non-fatal stroke decreased by 44% (p=0.007). In active treatment group, all fatal and non-fatal cardiac endpoints, including sudden death, declined by 26% (p=0.03). Non-fatal cardiac endpoints decreased by 33% (p=0.03) and all fatal and non-fatal CV endpoints by 31% (p<0.001). CV mortality was slightly lower on active treatment (-27%, p=0.07), but all-cause mortality was not influenced (-14%; p=0.22).

Ref: Lancet 1997; 350:757-64.

· HOT
Hypertension Optimal Treatment

> Intensive lowering of BP in patients with HT is associated with a low rate of CV events. Moreover, aspirin significantly reduces the major CV events.

In this study, 18,790 patients, from 26 countries, aged 50–80 years with HT and DBP 100-115 mmHg were randomly assigned a target DBP. 6264 patients were allocated to target pressure ⩽90, 6264 to ⩽85, and 6262 to ⩽80. Felodipine was given as baseline therapy with addition of other agents, according to a five-step regimen. In addition, these patients were randomly assigned 75 mg/day aspirin or placebo.

DBP was reduced by 20·3, 22·3, and 24·3 mmHg in ⩽90, ⩽85, and ⩽80 mmHg target groups, respectively. The lowest incidence of major CV events occurred at a mean achieved DBP 82·6 mmHg; the lowest risk of CV mortality occurred at 86·5. Further reduction below these BPs was safe. In patients with DM there was 51% reduction in major CV events in target group ⩽80 compared with ⩽90 (p for trend=0·005). Aspirin reduced major CV events by 15% (p=0·03) and all MI by 36% (p=0·002), with no effect on stroke. There were 7 fatal bleeds in aspirin group and 8 in placebo, and 129 versus 70 nonfatal major bleeds, respectively (p<0·001).

Ref: Lancet 1998; 351: 1755-62.

. DASH
Dietary Approaches to Stop Hypertension

> DASH diet, which is rich in fruits, vegetables, and low-fat dairy foods, significantly lowers the BP.

Among 459 participants, 72 had stage 1 isolated systolic HT (ISH) (SBP 140-159 mmHg; DBP <90 mmHg). After a 3-week run-in period on a typical American (control) diet, participants were randomly assigned for 8 weeks to 1 of the 3 diets: continuation of control diet (n=25), a diet rich in fruits and vegetables (n=24), or the DASH diet (n=23). Sodium content was same in the 3 diets, and caloric intake was adjusted during the trial to prevent the weight change. BP was measured at baseline and at the end of 8-week intervention period with standard sphygmomanometry.

DASH diet significantly lowered SBP compared with control diet (-11.2 mm Hg; 95% CI, -6.1 to -16.2 mmHg; P<0.001) and the fruits/vegetables diet (-8.0 mm Hg; 95% CI, -2.5 to -13.4 mmHg; P<0.01). Overall, BP in the DASH group fell from 146/85 to 134/82 mmHg. Similar results were observed with 24-hour ABPM. In DASH diet group, 18 of 23 participants (78%) reduced their systolic BP to <140 mmHg, compared with 24% and 50% in the control and fruits/vegetables groups, respectively.

Ref: Hypertension 2001; 38:155-8.

· CAPPP
Captopril Prevention Project

> Captopril and conventional treatment doesn't differ in efficacy in preventing the CV morbidity and mortality.

In this prospective, randomised, open trial with blinded endpoint evaluation, 10,985 patients were enrolled at 536 health centres in Sweden and Finland. Patients aged 25-66 years with a measured DBP $\geq$100 mmHg on two occasions were randomly assigned captopril or conventional antihypertensive treatment (diuretics, beta-blockers). The primary endpoint was a composite of fatal and non-fatal MI, stroke, and other CV deaths.

Primary end-point events occurred in 363 patients in captopril group (11.1 per 1000 patient-years) and 335 in conventional-treatment group (10.2 per 1000 patient-years; RR 1.05 [95% CI 0.90-1.22], p=0.52). CV mortality was lower with captopril than conventional treatment (76 vs 95 events; RR 0.77 [0.57-1-04], p=0.09), the rate of fatal and non-fatal MI was similar (162 vs 161), but fatal and non-fatal stroke was more common with captopril (189 vs 148; 1.25 [1-01-1-55]. p=0.04).

Ref: Lancet 1999; 353:611-6.

· AASK

African-American Study of Kidney disease and hypertension

> Ramipril, compared with amlodipine, retards the renal disease progression in patients with hypertensive renal disease and proteinuria and may offer benefit to patients without proteinuria.

In this RCT, 1094 African-Americans age 18-70 with hypertensive renal disease GFR 20-65 ml/min were randomly assigned to receive amlodipine, 5-10 mg/d, ramipril, 2.5-10 mg/d, or metoprolol, 50-200 mg/d, with other agents added to achieve 1 of 2 BP goals, on hypertensive renal disease progression. Participants were with urinary protein to creatinine ratio >0.22 (corresponding to proteinuria of >300 mg/d).

Ramipril group had a 36% (2.02 [SE, 0.74] mL/min/y) slower mean decline in GFR over 3 years (P=0.006) and 48% reduced risk of clinical end points vs amlodipine group (95% CI, 20%-66%). In the entire cohort, there was no significant difference in mean GFR decline from baseline to 3 years between treatment groups (P=0.38). However, compared with amlodipine group, after adjustment for baseline covariates ramipril group had 38% reduced risk of clinical end points (95% CI, 13%-56%), 36% slower mean decline in GFR after 3 months (P =.002), and less proteinuria (P<.001).

Ref: JAMA. 2001; 285:2719-28.

· HOPE
Heart Outcomes Prevention Evaluation

Ramipril significantly reduces the cardiovascular events (MI, stroke and death) in high-risk patients with normal ejection fraction.

A total of 9297 high-risk patients (>55 years) who had evidence of vascular disease or diabetes plus one other CV risk factor and who were not known to have low EF or heart failure were randomly assigned to receive ramipril (10 mg once a day) or matching placebo for a mean of five years. The primary outcome was a composite of MI, stroke, or death from CV causes. The trial was a two-by-two factorial study evaluating both ramipril and vitamin E.

A total of 651 patients who were assigned to receive ramipril (14%) reached the primary end-point, as compared with 826 patients assigned to placebo (17.8%) (RR, 0.78; 95%, 0.70 to 0.86; P<0.001). Treatment with ramipril significantly reduced the rates of death from CV causes, MI, stroke, death from any cause, revascularization procedures, cardiac arrest, heart failure, and complications related to diabetes.

Ref: N Engl J Med 2000; 342:145-53.

. ACCOMPLISH

Avoiding Cardiovascular events through COMbination therapy in Patients LIving with Systolic HT

ACE-I & CCB combination is superior to ACE-I plus thiazide in reducing the cardiovascular events in patients with HT who are at high risk for such events.

In this RCT, 11,506 patients with HT who were at high risk for CV events were randomized to receive either benazepril plus amlodipine or benazepril plus HCT.

The trial was terminated early after a mean follow-up of 36 months, when the boundary of prespecified stopping rule was exceeded.

Mean BP after dose adjustment was 131.6/73.3 mmHg in benazepril–amlodipine group and 132.5/74.4 mmHg in benazepril–HCT group.

There were 552 primary-outcome events in ACE-I/CCB group (9.6%) and 679 in ACE-I–HCT group (11.8%), representing an absolute RR with ACE-I/CCB therapy of 2.2% and RR reduction of 19.6% (hazard ratio, 0.80, 95% CI, 0.72 to 0.90; P<0.001). For the secondary end point of death from CV causes, nonfatal MI, and nonfatal stroke, the hazard ratio was 0.79 (95% CI, 0.67 to 0.92; P=0.002).

Ref: New Engl J Med 2008; 359:2417-28.

CHRONIC LIVER DISEASE

SUMMARY

This gentleman, Mr. Bakhsh, 55 years old, from D.I.Khan, is suffering from chronic HCV with cirrhosis. He gives past history of hospitalization for upper GI bleed a year age. After that event he had three sessions of endoscopic variceal band *ligation*. This time he presented with hematemesis and altered mental state 5 days back.

On examination he is pale, mildly jaundiced and has tense ascites. His liver is not palpable and spleen can be felt by dipping method 2 fingers beyond the left costal margin.

He has got:

Chronic HCV with Cirrhosis and its sequelae; Portal hypertension, Upper GI bleed and Hepatic encephalopathy.
He is now out of overt encephalopathy - West-Heaven score 1/6, has tense ascites and is hemodynamically stable after upper GI bleed.

MANAGEMENT PLAN

His acute problems; "Hepatic encephalopathy and Upper GI bleed" are now settled. I would have resuscitated the patient and arranged for an urgent OGD with possible intervention as required.

I will perform investigations like FBC, LFTs including S. albumin & PT, U&Es, S. creatinine.

I will calculate the Child Pugh and MELD score to assess the severity of underlying liver disease and estimate the prognosis.

I will perform diagnostic paracentesis to rule out SBP.

I will perform Anti-HCV, HBcAb, S. ferritin, and caeruloplasmin levels to rule out the important differentials for CLD.

I will prescribe prophylactic antibiotics for SBP (third generation parenteral cephalosporin).

I will prescribe lactulose for prophylaxis of PSE.

I will prescribe vasoactive drugs such as Terlipressin or Somatostatin analogue for possible variceal bleed.

I will arrange for an early endoscopy and treatment for varices like band ligation or sclerotherapy.

I will prescribe blood transfusion if Hb < 7g/dl.

I will admit the patient and refer to the Gastro/Liver unit after acute initial management and stabilization.

Later on he may need appropriate antiviral therapy for HCV after doing PCR, viral load and genotyping.

I will arrange for abdominal USG $\pm$ AFP to screen for HCC.

I will arrange for GP appointment at 2 weeks and specialist appointment at 4 weeks on discharge from the hospital.

DISCUSSION

After mentioning the initial stabilization ABC and 2S (Supportive and Symptomatic interventions), the discussion may revolve around the management and diagnostic aspects of the following conditions:

- Cirrhosis liver

- Acute variceal bleed

- Hepatic encephalopathy

Up-to-date knowledge regarding these topics can be obtained from various sources available online like:

http://www.easl.eu

http://www.bsg.org.uk

http://www.aasld.org

Some tips to tackle the discussion successfully are given in the following pages.

CIRRHOSIS LIVER

C irrhosis liver is due to fibrosis and regeneration of liver cells in response to hepatocellular injury, leading to liver cell dysfunction, portal hypertension and their sequelae.

Clinically it is classified as "Compensated" or "Decompensated".

It is labeled as decompensated when there is jaundice, variceal bleed, encephalopathy, or ascites.

CAUSES

- Alcohol: The most common cause in the Western world.
- Viral hepatitis: Chronic HBV, HCV; the most common cause in the Asia.
- Autoimmune hepatitis: More common in females.
- Metabolic: Hemochromatosis, Wilson's disease, α-1 anti-trypsin deficiency.
- Biliary tract disease: Primary biliary cholangitis (PBC), Primary sclerosing cholangitis (PSC).
- Vascular disease: Budd-Chiari syndrome, CCF, Constrictive pericarditis, Sinusidal obstructive syndrome
- Non-alcoholic fatty liver disease (NAFLD)
- Cryptogenic

GRADING

◆ Child-Pugh Score:

It predicts the prognosis in CLD and cirrhosis.

CHILD PUGH SCORE

Factor	1 point	2 points	3 points
S. bilirubin (mg/dl)	<2	2-3	>3
S. albumin (g/dl)	>3.5	2.8-3.5	<2.8
INR	<1.7	1.7-2.3	>2.3
Ascites	None	Mild	Moderate to severe
Hepatic encephalopathy	None	Grade I-II (or suppressed with medication)	Grade III-IV (or refractory)

Grading	Class A	Class B	Class C
Total points	5-6	7-9	10-15
1-year survival	100%	80%	45%

◆ MELD Score
(Model for End-stage Liver Disease)

It is a reliable measure of mortality risk in patients with end-stage liver disease. It is used to stratify the patients on liver transplant list for priority.

$$\text{MELD} = 3.78 \times \text{Bilirubin (mg/dl)} + 11.2 \times \text{INR} + 9.57 \times \text{Creatinine (mg/dl)} + 6.4$$

If the patient was dialysed twice within the last 7 days, then creatinine is taken as 4 mg/dl. Any value less than 1 is rounded (e.g. bilirubin 0.8 is taken as 1).

Interpretation:	Score	Mortality
	≥40	71.3%
	30-39	52.6%
	20-29	19.6%
	10-19	6%
	<19	1.9%

COMPLICATIONS

F ollowing are the important complications responsible for the morbidity and mortality of patients with CLD.

Acute variceal bleed

Hepatic encephalopathy

Subacute bacterial peritonitis

Hepatocellular carcinoma

Each of these complications will be discussed in the fol-low-ing sections.

ASCITES

P athological accumulation of fluid in the peritoneal cavity. It is the most common complication of cirrhosis; 50% of patients develop ascites within 10 years of diagnosis. Ascites has significant impact on the patient health by frequent hospitalization, leading to complications like SBP and hepatorenal syndrome.

PATHOPHYSIOLOGY

Ascites is the result of a series of anatomic, pathophysio-logic and biochemical abnormalities.

Portal hypertension: The first step towards fluid retention is the development of portal HT; portal pressure >12 mmHg is required for fluid retention.

Vasodilatation: In cirrhosis progressive vasodilatation is observed primarily due to increased nitric oxide release, which leads to activation of endogenous vaso-constriction, sodium and water retention and increasing renal vasoconstriction. The vasodilatation results in activation of sodium-retaining neurohumoral mechanisms in an attempt to restore perfusion pressure to normal. These include renin-angiotensin-aldosterone system, sympathetic nervous system, and antidiuretic hormone (vasopressin). The net effect is sodium and water retention.

EVALUATION & DIAGNOSIS

Ascites can be uncomplicated, infected, refractory or associated with renal impairment.

It is graded based on the amount of fluid.

- **Grade 1 (Mild):** Only detectable by USG.
- **Grade 2 (Moderate):** Moderate, symmetrical distension of abdomen.
- **Grade 3 (Gross):** Marked abdominal distension.

Diagnostic paracentesis: It is indicated in;

- All patients with new onset grade 2 or 3 ascites.
- Patients hospitalized for worsening ascites or any complication of cirrhosis.

In ascitic fluid analysis the following should be noted;

Neutrophil count and culture: To exclude bacterial peritonitis. Neutrophil count >250 cells/μl denotes SBP.

Protein concentration: To identify patients at higher risk of developing SBP.

SAAG: Should be calculated when the cause of ascites is not evident or conditions other than cirrhosis are suspected.

Cytology: To differentiate malignant from non-malignant ascites.

ALGORYTHM FOR THE DIAGNOSTIC WORK-UP IN ASCITES

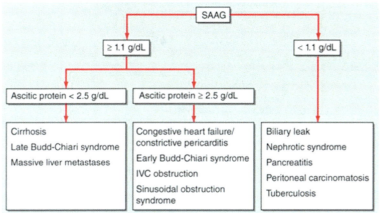

MANAGEMENT

The goals of management are:
- Treatment of the underlying disease
- Treatment of ascites
- Prevention of complications
- Treatment of complications

UNCOMPLICATED ASCITES

The treatment of ascites in cirrhosis includes abstinence from alcohol, dietary sodium restriction, and diuretics.

Patients with tense ascites should undergo an initial therapeutic paracentesis.

Grade 1 (Mild): No data on evolution and not known if treatment modifies the natural history.

Grade 2 (Moderate): Moderate dietary sodium restriction (80-120 mmol/day, 4.6-6.9 g of salt) and diuretics. Gener-ally, equivalent to diet with no added salt and avoidance of pre-prepared meals.

Grade 3 (Massive): Large volume paracentesis (LVP) is the treatment of choice.

Ascites can be completely removed in single session. LVP should be followed by plasma volume expansion by albu-min infusion (8 g per litre of ascites removed).

After LVP patients should receive minimum dose of diuret-ics necessary to prevent re-accumulation. Before starting diuretic therapy the following conditions should be cor-rected: Upper GI bleed, renal impairment, hepatic en-cephalopathy and electrolytes imbalance.

Anti-mineralocorticoid drugs are the mainstay of diuretic therapy, loop diuretics may be added in patients with long standing ascites.

In first episode of grade 2 ascites only anti-mineralocorticoid (spironolactone) should be given (100 mg/day with 100 mg stepwise increase every 72 hrs, max. 400 mg/day).

In patients who don't respond to spironolactone or devel-op hyperkalaemia, furosemide should be added (40 mg/day maximum 160 mg/day).

In long-standing or recurrent ascites, combination of spi-ronolactone and furosemide is given in a ratio of 100:40.

Monitoring of patients on diuretics:

Frequent clinical and biochemical assessment should be performed as these patients are highly susceptible to rapid reduction in extracellular fluid volume leading to renal failure.

Response to diuretics is assessed by weight loss. Recommended maximum weight loss is 0.5 kg/day in patients without and 1 kg/day with peripheral edema.

Once ascites has largely resolved, the dose of diuretics should be reduced to the lowest effective dose. Discontin-ue diuretics in severe hyponatremia, AKI, worsening HE, or incapacitating muscle cramps.

REFRACTORY ASCITES

International Ascites Club defines refractory ascites as the one that cannot be mobilized or early recurrence after LVP can't be satisfactorily prevented by medical therapy. It has two type.

Diuretic resistant: Ascites that cannot be mobilized or early recurrence can't be prevented because of lack of response to sodium restriction and diuretic treat-ment.

Diuretic intractable: Ascites that cannot be mobilized or early recurrence can't be prevented because of development of diuretic-induced complications that preclude the use of effective diuretic dosage.

Repeated LVP plus albumin: Albumin 8 g per litre of asci-tes removed is recommended as the first-line treatment.

Diuretics should be discontinued in patients with refractory ascites who do not excrete >30 mmol/day of sodium on diuretic treatment.

NSBBs: Controversial data exist on the use of NSBBs in refractory ascites, caution should be exercised in severe cases. High doses should be avoided (like propranolol >80 mg/day).

TIPS: Patients should be evaluated for TIPS when other measures mentioned fail.

TIPS

P atients should be evaluated for TIPS when there is refractory or recurrent ascites and paracentesis is ineffective. It improves the control of ascites and survival.

After TIPS, continue diuretics and salt restriction and close clinical follow-up until ascites resolution.

CONTRAINDICATIONS

Absolute:

- Severe CHF
- Severe pulmonary HT
- Polycystic liver disease
- Severe hepatic failure
- Portal Vein thrombosis with cavernoma formation

Relative:

- Active infection
- Poorly controlled PSE
- Hypervascular liver tumor
- Portal vein thrombosis without carvernoma
- Biliary obstruction

ACUTE VARICEAL BLEED

V aricial bleed is the most common cause of death in patients with cirrhosis. Mortality during the first episode is 15-30% or even higher in patients with severe disease. Patients with cirrhosis presenting with upper GI bleed have varices as the source of bleeding in 50-90% cases while a variety of other causes like gastric ulceration can also occur.

MANAGEMENT

It requires multidisciplinary approach involving Hepa-tolo-gist, Intensive Care Specialist, Surgeon and Inter-ventional Radiologist.

Initial resuscitation

Pre-endoscopic pharmacologic therapy

Endoscopic management

INITIAL RESUSCITATION

Patients should preferably be managed at HDU.

The most important step in the management is initial resuscitation according to the standard "ABC" practice.

The airway should be protected to prevent aspir-ation.

In patients with massive bleed endotracheal intubation can be considered to protect the airways.

IV access with two large bore cannulae (18 G).

IV fluid should be initiated with plasma expanders aiming to maintain SBP 100 mmHg.

Patients must be monitored carefully to avoid over transfusion with volume overload because of the risk of rebound portal HT and rebleed.

Platelets transfusion when count <50 x109/L.

FFP if fibrinogen level <1 g/L or INR >1.5.

PRE-ENDOSCOPIC THERAPY

Antibiotics:

IV erythromycin (single dose, 250 mg 30–120 minutes prior to upper GI endoscopy) in patients with clinically severe or ongoing active bleed significantly improves the endoscopic visualization, reduces the need for second-look endoscopy, units of blood transfused and hospital stay.

Contraindications to erythromycin include sensitivity to macrolides and prolonged QT interval.

Prophylactic antibiotics reduce the risk of re-bleed, infec-tious complications and mortality. Third-generation cepha-losporin, such as ceftriaxone have been shown to be effec-tive at reducing Gram-negative sepsis but the choice of antibiotics should be dictated by local antibiotic policy.

Vasoactive drugs:

Vasopressin (or its analogue terlipressin) and somatostatin (or its analogue octreotide)

These should be started as soon as possible and continued until hemostasis is achieved or up to 5 days.

Vasopressin reduces portal blood flow, portal-systemic collateral blood flow and variceal pressure. The recommended dose of terlipressin is 2 mg IV every 4 h, although many centers reduce the dose to 6 hourly as it may cause peripheral vasoconstriction which manifests as painful hands and feet. Significant side effects include increase in peripheral resistance and decreased cardiac output; so it should not be used in high cardiovascular-risk patients.

Somatostatin causes selective splanchnic vasoconstriction and reduces the portal pressure and portal blood flow. Octreotide (a somatostatin analogue) is given as 50 μg bolus followed by infusion of 25–50 μg/h.

Lactulose:

It is given to prevent HE. Can be given orally or rectally as enema if the patient is vomiting.

Note: There is no role of PPIs in the management of variceal bleed.

NG tube is not routinely recommended in the management of variceal bleed.

ENDOSCOPIC THERAPY

All patients with suspected variceal bleed should undergo OGD within 12 hours after initial resuscitation. There are two techniques for its management.

- Band ligation
- Sclerotherpay

Band ligation:

It is a modification of elastic band ligation for internal hemorrhoids. It works by capturing all or part of a varix resulting in occlusion from thrombosis. The tissue then gets necrosed and sloughs-off in days to weeks, leaving a superficial mucosal ulceration, which rapidly heals.

Repeated every 2-4 weeks till the obliteration of varices.

Minor complications can occur such as dysphagia or chest pain. Post-banding ulcer bleeding is a rare complication.

Sclerotherapy:

It is the oldest endoscopic treatment for variceal bleed. Due to formation of ulcer on the site of injection, sometimes responsible for hemorrhage, sclero-therapy should be abandoned.

Sclerotherpay is done with tissue adhesives most commonly histoacryl (N-butyl-cyanoacrylate) for fundal varices. Initial hemostasis success rate with tissue glue is 86–100%, with re-bleed rates of 7–28% is reported.

Uncommon, but serious complications include pulmonary or cerebral embolism.

EVL has been compared to sclerotherapy in several studies; all showing lesser rebleed and fewer side effects with EVL.

Failure of Endoscopic Therapy:

Failure to control active bleeding is defined by one of the following criteria:

☐ Fresh hematemesis or NG aspiration of ≥100 ml fresh blood ≥2 h after the start of a specific drug treatment or therapeutic endoscopy.

☐ Development of hypovolemic shock.

☐ 3 g/dl drop in Hb (9% drop of hematocrit) within 24 hours if no transfusion is given.

In case of failure of endoscopic therapy the following op-tions can be tried:

Balloon tamponade

Removable esophageal stent

TIPS

Porto-systemic surgical shunts

Liver transplant

PROPHYLAXIS

Primary:

Non-selective β-blocker (propranolol, nadolol, carvedilol) or band ligation.

Secondary:

Non-selective β-blocker and band ligation.

HEPATIC ENCEPHALOPATHY

H epatic encephalopathy (HE) is a potentially re- versible brain dysfunction caused by liver in- sufficiency &/or porto-systemic shunting. It manifests as a wide spectrum of neurologic and psychiatric abnor- malities ranging from subclinical alterations to coma.

HE occurs due to a combination of distinct pathophysiological mechanisms such as inflammation, oxidative stress, impaired blood-brain barrier perme- ability, neurotoxins, impaired energy metabolism of brain and more.

Overt HE develops in 30-45% of patients with cirrho- sis during their clinical course. Minimal or covert HE occurs in 20-80% patients with cir-rhosis.

CLINICAL MANIFESTATIONS

HE produces a wide spectrum of nonspecific neuro- logical and psychiatric manifestations.

In minimal or covert HE cognitive findings are very subtle, not apparent without specialized testing. As the disease progresses the changes become more overt with impair-ments in attention, reaction time and working memory. Severe cases may progress to coma.

Disturbances in the diurnal sleep pattern (insomnia and hypersomnia) are the common initial manifest- ations.

Neuromuscular impairment in patients with overt

HE includes bradykinesia, asterixis (flapping motions of out-stretched, dorsiflexed hands), slurred speech, ataxia, hy-peractive deep tendon reflexes, and nystagmus. Motor system abnormalities includes hypertonia, hyper-reflexia, and positive Babinski sign.

Focal neurological deficits are rare and seizures very rare.

PRECIPITANTS

GI bleed

Infection

Electrolyte imbalance(↓ K)

High protein diet

Diuretic overdose

Renal impairment

Hypovolemia

Hypoxia

Sedative drugs

Hypoglycemia

Constipation

Hepatocellular carcinoma

CLASSIFICATION

According to the underlying disease:

Type A: Resulting from acute liver failure

Type B: Predominantly from portosystemic bypass or shunting

Type C: Resulting from cirrhosis

According to severity of manifestations:

Covert: Minimal - Grade 1

Overt: Grade 2-4

According to its time course:

Episodic:

Recurrent: Bouts of HE that occur with a time interval of 6 months or less.

Persistent: A pattern of behavioral alteration that is always present and interspersed with relapses of overt HE.

According to the existence of precipitating factors:

Spontaneous

Precipitated

STAGING

There are various scoring systems to grade HE. The commonly used one is West-Haven system also called Conn score.

WEST-HAVEN CLASSIFICATION OF HEPATIC ENCEPHALOPATHY

Stage	Features
0	No abnormality detected
I	Trivial lack of awareness, euphoria or anxiety, shortened attention span, impairment of addition or subtraction
II	Lethargy or apathy, disorientation for time, obvious personality change, inappropriate behavior
III	Somnolence to semistupor, responsive to stimuli, confused, gross disorientation, bizarre behavior
IV	Coma, unable to test mental state

DIAGNOSIS

The approach to the diagnosis includes:

☐ History and physical exam to detect the cognitive and neuromuscular impairments that characterize HE.

☐ Exclusion of other causes of mental status changes.

☐ Evaluation for possible precipitating causes.

☐ Laboratory testing: Raised blood-ammonia level.

CT/MRI brain or other image modality do not contribute diagnostic or grading information. However, the risk of intracerebral hemorrhage is 5-fold increased in these pa-tients and as the symptoms may be indistinguishable, so a brain scan may be required.

MANAGEMENT

Identification and correction of precipitating causes

Measures to lower blood NH3 concentration:

- Proteins restriction
- Lactulose /lactitol
- Rifaximin

Lactulose is a non-absorbable disaccharides having following beneficial effects.

It acidifies the colon which converts NH3 to NH4+, trapping NH4+ in the colon thus reducing plasma ammonia concentration.

It is also a laxative and has prebiotic effects (the drug being a non-digestible substance, promotes the growth of beneficial microorganisms in the intestines).

Oral antibiotics have role in reducing blood ammonia levels and are used as add on therapy to disaccharides. Rifaximin is currently used most often; 550 mg PO BD or 400 mg TDS. It ↓ bacteria and thus NH3 production.

Neomycin was widely used in the past. It has variable efficacy and with prolonged use there are concerns of oto and nephrotoxicity.

As short-term therapy, metronidazole also has advocates for its use. However, long-term oto, nephro, and neurotoxicity make it unattractive for long-term use.

There are some other agents with questionable efficacy in the management of HE. These can be tried as add-on therapy when conventional approach fails.

L-ornithine-L-aspartate (LOLA)

Branched-chain amino acids

Prebiotics and probiotics

Nutrition in hepatic encephalopathy:

Daily energy intakes should be 35-40 kcal/kg body wt. and protein intake 1.2-1.5 g/kg.

Small meals or liquid nutritional supplements evenly dis-tributed throughout the day and a late-night snack should be offered.

PREVENTION

☐ Avoid precipitants

☐ Lactulose

☐ Lactulose + Rifaximine

Prophylactic therapy (lactulose or rifaximin) is recommended only for secondary prevention; not for primary prevention.

ROLE OF RIFAXIMIN
IN HEPATIC ENCEPHALOPATHY

Rifaximin is a broad spectrum, locally acting, oral antibi-otic used both in the secondary prevention and treatment of HE.

It reduces the colonic ammonia (NH_3) absorption by de-creasing the population of urease producing bacteria in the large gut.

SPONTANEOUS BACTERIAL PERITONITIS

S pontaneous bacterial peritonitis (SBP) is defined as bacterial infection of ascitic fluid without any intra-abdominal, surgically treatable source of infection. The prevalence of SBP ranges from 1.5% to 3.5% in out-patient and 10% in hospitalized patients.

Patients with cirrhosis are at increased risk of bacterial infections due to a number of reasons:
- Liver dysfunction
- Porto-systemic shunting
- Gut dysbiosis
- Blood transfusions
- Cirrhosis-associated immune dysfunction

Previously the mortality of SBP was around 90% but now due to early diagnosis and prompt treatment with antibi-otics it has reduced to 20%.

DIAGNOSIS

Diagnosis of SBP is based on the results of paracentesis.

The patients may present with a wide range of clinical symptoms including abdominal pain & tenderness, vomit-ing, diarrhea, worsening of ascites, fever, hepatic encephalopathy or upper GI bleed. SBP can have asymptomatic presentation especially in out-patients.

Diagnostic paracentesis should be carried out in patients with:

☐ At time of hospital admission in cirrhotic patients with ascites.

☐ All patients presenting with worsening of ascites, upper GI bleed, fever, hepatic encephalopathy and deranged renal function.

Diagnostic paracentesis should include biochemical analy-sis, total cell count with differential and ascitic fluid cul-ture.

SBP is diagnosed when neutrophil count of ascetic fluid is >250/mm³.

The positive ascitic fluid culture can add to the diagnosis but it is not the prerequisite.
There are two types of SBP.
Classical SBP: Neutrophil count >250/mm3 and positive culture.
Culture negative neutrocytic ascites: Neutrophil >250/mm³ and negative culture.

Bacteriology of SBP:
-    Gram negative bacilli   70%
        Escherichia coli
        Klebsiella spp.
-    Gram positive cocci   20%
        Streptococcus pneumonae
        Enterococcus spp.

Staphylococcus spp.

- Anaerobes, Microaerophils & others   10%

MANAGEMENT

Empirical IV antibiotics should be started soon after the diagnosis.

In community acquired SBP third generation ceph-alospor-ins are recommended as first line agents especially in countries with low rates of antibiotic resistance.

In hospital acquired SBP piperacillin/tazobactam or carbapenem are recommended.

If culture of ascitic fluid is positive, titrate the antibiotics accordingly. The duration of treatment is 5-7 days.

The efficacy of antibiotics is checked by repeating paracen-tesis after 48 hrs. Failure of first-line agents is suspected if worsening of clinical symptoms, increase or no decrease in neutrophil count (at least 25%).

Two doses of salt-free albumin are recommended: One on the day of diagnosis (1.5 g/kg), and another on 3rd day (1.0 g/kg).

PROPHYLAXIS

Primary: It is recommended with norfloxacin 400 mg once-a-day in patients with:

Child score >9 and serum bilirubin >3 mg/dl, either impaired renal function or hyponaterima and ascitic fluid protein <15 g/L.

The drug should be stopped with long-lasting clinical improvement or disappearance of ascites.

Secondary: Secondary prophylaxis is recommended in patients who survived the first episode with norfloxacin 400 mg once a day.

These patients have poor long-term survival so they should be considered for liver transplant.

HEPATOCELLULAR CARCINOMA

Hepatocellular carcinoma (HCC) is the most common pri-mary malignancy of the liver. Its incidence is highest in Asia and Africa due to the high prevalence of hepatitis B and C. It develops in 3-8% of patients with chronic HBV or HCV per year.

RISK FACTORS

- Cirrhosis liver of any etiology

- Chronic hepatitis B and C

- Alcoholic liver disease

- Non-alcoholic fatty liver disease (NFLD)

- Hemochromatosis

- Aflatoxin exposure

- Obesity and diabetes mellitus

- Rare inherited disorders like glycogen storage disease, alpha-1 antitrypsin deficiency, metal storage disease and chronic cholestatic syndromes.

CLINICAL FEATURES

HCC may be asymptomatic or the patient may present with hepatic decompensation (ascites, encephalopathy), or portal vein thrombosis.

DIAGNOSIS

Mainly based on the imaging studies and biochemical marker AFP without the need for biopsy.

Imaging:

All cirrhotic patients are routinely screened for HCC by doing USG every 6 months with or without AFP.

If a liver nodule <1 cm is detected on USG, repeat after 3 months. If >1 cm with AFP >20 ng/ml then further imaging is advised with either multiphasic CT or dynamic contrast enhanced MRI.

Due to the differential blood supply of HCC as compared to the background liver the lesion appears brighter on arterial phase and less bright than the rest of the liver in venous phase (arterial enhancement and delayed washout), the radiological hallmark of HCC, no further testing is advised for diagnosis.

Alpha Fetoprotein:

A biochemical marker for HCC used for the diagnosis and monitoring of treatment. Patients with cirrhosis should be screened every 6 months with AFP and abdominal USG.

Biopsy:

If atypical features of the lesion are seen on imaging then biopsy and histopathologic examination is advised.

GALAD score:
It is a statistical model for estimating the likelihood of HCC in patients with CLD and their survival.

It combines the patient demographics (gender and age) with serum biomarkers AFP, AFP-L3, and Desgamma carboxy prothrombin (DCP).

Web-based calculators are available to quickly determine the GALAD score:

http://www.mayoclinic.org/medical-professionals/model-end-stage-liver-disease/gala

SCREENING
The outcome in HCC primarily depends upon its detection in the earlier stages. For this reason HCC screening is ad-vised in high risk population including patients with liver cirrhosis and sub group of patients with chronic HBV, Asian male, age >40 years, family history of HCC.

International societies recommend screening for HCC eve-ry 6 monthly with USG of abdomen.

The data suggest that USG is an operator dependent modality and performance is affected by factors like obesity, ascites and fatty infiltrates of the liver.

Several biomarker are present for HCC but the most

stud-ied and validated one is AFP. Meta-analysis has shown that combining AFP with USG has increased the detection ratio of HCC among high risk population.

Surveillance with CT/MRI may increase the sensitivity for early detection of HCC but there are concerns such as ra-diation exposure, contrast exposure and cost implications.

MANAGEMENT

The decision about selection of treatment modality depends upon three factors:

- Tumor characteristics (number & size, vascular invasion, distant metastasis)
- Functional status of the patient (according to ECOG)
- Child Pugh class of patient

After getting above mentioned information the patient is staged according to the "Barcelona Clinic for Liver Cancer" (BCLC) staging system and the treatment modality is selected.

Resection:

Suitable for a solitary lesion <2 cm in a patient with Child-Pugh A cirrhosis without portal hy-pertension.

Radiofrequency ablation (RFA):

Suitable for multifocal HCC with lesions <3 cm in size.

Transarterial chemo-embolization (TACE):

Preferred for large lesions (not with curative intent) or small le-sions but not amenable to RFA (like lesion near IVC).

Liver transplant:

For liver transplantation of HCC patients in addition to BCLC staging system, Milan criteria is also used.

It is the best option if up to 3 lesions ≤3 cm or a single lesion ≤5 cm. The results of liver transplantation are very encouraging with 5 year survival of 70% and 10 year survival 50%. Recurrence rates are 10-15% at 5 years.

Tyrosine kinase inhibitors:

To bridge the patients up to the liver transplant and to delay the recurrence.

BARCELONA CLINIC FOR LIVER CANCER (BCLC) STAGING SYSTEM

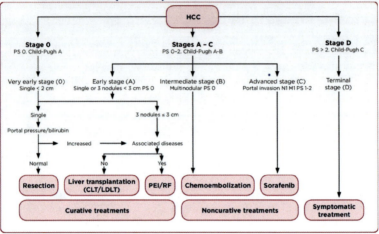

EASTERN CO-OPERATIVE ONCOLOGY GROUP (ECOG) FUNCTIONAL STATUS

0: Fully active, able to carry on all pre-disease performance without restriction.

1: Restriction in physically strenuous activity but ambulatory and able to carry out work of light nature.

2: Ambulatory and capable of all self-care but unable to carry out any work activities. Up and about more than 50% of waking hours.

3: Capable of only limited self-care, confined to bed or chair more than 50% of waking hours.

4: Completely disabled can't carry on self-care. Totally confined to bed or chair.

5: Dead.

PROGNOSIS

The overall prognosis of HCC is poor with 5 year survival rate of 18.4%.

By stage, the 5 year survival is 32.6% for localized disease, 10.8% with regional disease, and 2.4% for metastatic disease.

LAND-MARK TRIALS

◆ ENDOSCOPIC ESOPHAGEAL VARIX LIGATION

This study established the endoscopic variceal ligation as a safe and effective treatment for esophageal varices.

This was the first ever published trial in which esophageal variceal band ligation was done, which later became the standard of care endoscopic management of varices. Before this trial injection sclerotherapy was done which had the risk of serious side effects and less success rate.

In this trial EVL was performed in 14 patients who had recently bled from esophageal varices. None was actively bleeding at the initial treatment.

There were no procedural complications. 132 varix ligations were performed in 44 sessions. Two patients were lost to follow-up and two died; neither death resulted from hemorrhage or treatment complications. Variceal rebleeding occurred in 2 noncompliant patients (14.3%) and was successfully controlled with emergent EVL. Ten patients achieved complete variceal eradication with 1-6 (mean, 3.9) sessions. No major complications (perforation, secondary bleeding, deep ulceration) resulted and there were no treatment failures. Follow-up of 10 surviving patients ranged from 240-370 (mean, 280) days. Endoscopic observation suggested that varices were obliterated by a process of mechanical strangulation, ischemia, superficial ulceration, and scar formation.

Ref: Gastrointestinal Endoscopy 1998; 34;113-7.

◆ LIVER TRANSPLANTATION

Patients having liver transplantation show greater survival compared to those who did not undergo transplantation, permitting the establishment of liver transplant as a beneficial procedure for end-stage liver disease.

A series of 540 cases united by 4 different liver transplant units was presented at the 1983 NIH Conference.

After extensive review and consideration of all available data, this panel concludes that liver transplantation is a therapeutic modality for endstage liver disease that deserves broader application. However, in order for liver transplantation to gain its full therapeutic potential, the indications for and results of the procedure must be the object of comprehensive, coordinated, and ongoing evaluation in the years ahead. This can best be achieved by expansion of this technology to a limited number of centers where liver transplantation can be carried out under optimal conditions.

Ref: Hepatology 1984; 4(1 Suppl):107S-110S.

◆ BCLC STAGING

> The BCLC staging system was proposed to offer the best means of stage classification and treatment guidance for HCC.

Classifications of HCC currently used are based on prognostic factors obtained from studies performed years ago when most tumors were diagnosed at advanced stages and the survival rates were substantially poor. Recent investigations have reviewed the survival of early tumors properly selected to receive radical therapies and the natural outcome of nonsurgical HCC patients. These data enable a new staging system to be proposed, the Barcelona Clinic Liver Cancer (BCLC) staging classification that comprises four stages that select the best candidates for the best therapies currently available.

Early stage (A): Patients with asymptomatic early tumors suitable for radical therapies - resection, transplantation or percutaneous treatments.

Intermediate stage (B): Patients with asymptomatic multinodular HCC.

Advanced stage (C): Patients with symptomatic tumors &/or an invasive tumoral pattern (vascular invasion/extrahepatic spread).

Stage B and C patients may receive palliative treatments /new agents in the setting of phase II investigations or RCTs.

End-stage disease (D): Patients with extremely grim prognosis (Okuda stage III or PST 3-4) should merely receive symptomatic treatment.

Ref: Semin Liver Dis 1999; 19:329-38.

CEREBROVASCULAR DISEASE

P atients having cerebrovascular disease (CVD) like stroke can be brought forward as long-cases in the clinical exams because of their easy availability and because most of these patients have DM, HT &/or IHD as well. These additional co-morbidities make them a good case for discussion.

The summary and management plan of a typical case with stroke is given below.

SUMMARY

Mr. Chaudhry, a 65 years gentleman, known to have type 2 diabetes and HT for more than 10 years, presented with five days history of sudden-onset right-sided body weakness and difficulty in speaking.

On examination his pulse is 88 beats/min, irregularly-irregular, and BP 140/95 mmHg on medications. He has bilateral audible carotid bruits.

Auscultation of his heart revealed no abnormal findings except for the irregular and fast heart rate with pulsus deficit (heart rate faster than pulse rate).

Chest and abdomen examination are unremarkable.

Neurologic examination revealed a fully conscious gentleman having expressive dysphasia, right UMN facial weakness and right hemiparesis (power 4/5 on MRC scale, 0-5) with signs of UMN lesion i.e. hypertonia, hyper-reflexia, and extensor plantar response.

My diagnosis is:
Left hemispheric stroke likely cardio-embolic due to AF as presented with right hemiparesis, right facial UMN palsy, expressive dysphasia and irregularly-irregular pulse.

He is known to have type 2 diabetes and HT.

MANAGEMENT PLAN

This patient is already stable, however in the A&E, I would have taken care of the ABC, and requested an urgent CT scan or MRI of the brain.

Assessment by Rosier scale and imaging studies for timely thrombolysis or mechanical thrombectomy is important.

An ECG to confirm AF, and perform bed-side blood sugar to rule out hypoglycemia as a stroke mimic.

Later, I will request certain investigations like FBC, U&Es, lipid profile, HbA1c, INR and urinalysis.

I will also request carotid doppler study.

For diabetes, I will prescribe anti-diabetics after discussing with him the pros and cons of various antidiabetic agents, preferably "Physiologic SC scale insulin" while he is in the hospital.

For HT, I would like to prescribe a combination of CCB and ACE-I/ARB.

I will identify and manage the risk factors and predisposing conditions like smoking, dyslipidemia and AF in this case.

In the long run other important measures for a patient with stroke are Physiotherapy, Occupational therapy and Rehabilitation.

I would like to arrange a meeting with the Occupational therapist, Physiotherapist, Social worker, and Community nurse before his discharge from the hospital. Preferably, part-time home visits of the patient can also be arranged before his discharge.

At discharge, I will arrange for an early GP appointment and specialist clinic after 4 weeks' time.

DISCUSSION

As usual, the discussion will mainly revolve around the diagnostic and management aspects of stroke.

Some hints are given below to answer the possible questions.

Be prepared; the questions regarding DM, HT, or dyslipidemia can also be asked.

CEREBROVASCULAR DISEASE

S troke is a clinical syndrome defined by WHO as rapidly developed clinical signs of focal (sometimes global) disturbance of cerebral function, lasting longer than 24 hours or leading to death, with no apparent cause other than of vascular origin.

In acute ischemic stroke, time is critical and early management is the key to optimize the outcome.

Broadly, stroke can be ischemic in 80-85%, while hemorrhagic in 15-20% cases. It is more common in the males.

It is the 5th leading cause of death and the leading cause

of adult disability; the major cause of morbidity and mortality in elderly.

Classically, transient ischemic attack (TIA) is defined as sudden onset, focal neurological deficit or retinal ischemia, lasting less than 24 hours, presumed to be vascular in origin.

Focal neurological defecit of vascular origin that lasts >24 hours but recovers within a week, is sometimes called "minor stroke" or "reversible ischemic neurologic deficit" (RIND).

A neurological deficit that progresses or fluctuates while the patient is under observation, usually in the first 24 hours, is labeled as "stroke in evolution".

RISK FACTORS

Non-modifiable:

- Age: Stroke is uncommon before the age of 40.
- Gender: More common in males.
- Race/Ethnicity: Common in Afro-Caribbeans in UK.
- Family history

Modifiable:

The most common modifiable risk factors are DM, HT, dyslipidemia and smoking.

Others are:

- Heart and vascular disease (arteriosclerosis)
- Alcohol
- Oral contraceptives
- Obesity
- Sedentary life style

PREDISPOSING CONDITIONS

- Extra-cranial atheroma: Carotid /vertebral
- Intra-cranial atheroma
- Heart disease: AF (associated with 4 to 5-fold increase in the risk for ischemic stroke), valvular heart disease, recent MI, infective endocarditis
- Low cerebral perfusion: Hypotension due to any cause
- Hyperviscosity, Polycythemia
- Hypercoagulobility: Anti-phospholipid syndrome
- Arterial dissection: Carotid /vertebral
- Patent foramen ovale (PFO): Embolic /cortical stroke without any apparent cause other than moderately large PFO.
- CNS arteritis /vasculitis
- Moyamoya disease
- Metabolic disorders: MELAS, homocystinuria
- CADASIL (Cerebral autosomal dominant arteriopathy with subcortical infarcts and leuko-encephalopathy.
- Fabry's disease
- Sickle cell disease
- Bleeding disorders, anticoagulants Thrombolytics, antiplaletets.
- Berry aneurysms or AVM: For SAH

An interesting case history of a patient with stroke is presented below showing most of the risk factors for stroke.

Case History:

An interesting case history is presented below showing most of the risk factors for stroke.

A 68 years old, male shopkeeper, who remains on the shop from dawn to the dusk, presented with sudden onset right-sided weakness and inability to speak properly. He is known to have type 2 diabetes, and had a heart attack, and TIA in the past. He smokes two packs of cigarettes and drinks more than 2 units daily.

On examination, his pulse was 78 beats/min, irregularly-irregular and BP 210/120 mmHg. He had right hemiplegia with signs of UMN lesion. Examination of the face revealed left 3rd nerve palsy.

Blood tests revealed high total cholesterol level with high LDL-C & Triglycerides and carotid doppler revealed atheroma at the origin of left internal carotid artery.

- What is the diagnosis?
- Identify twelve risk factors or predisposing conditions for stroke present in this gentleman?
- Why this patient will need an urgent MRI rather than CT scan of the brain for proper management?
- Is there any role of anticoagulants in the management of this patient?

WARNING SIGNS

◆ FAST Test

Act fast - "Time is brain."

Early warning signs of acute stroke are important to recognize for the prompt action. FAST test is mainly meant for the general public and ambulance crew.

This will make the timely thrombolysis possible in "brain attack" just like "heart attack".

◆ ROSIER Scale

Recognition Of Stroke In Emergency Room

FAST test is used for public awareness and ambulance crew to identify acute stroke and take the patient immediately to the nearest hospital for further management.

While ROSIER scale is used in the ER to quickly recognize the stroke.

WARNING SIGNS FOR STROKE

F	**Face drooping**	
A	**Arm weakness**	
S	**Speech difficulty**	
T	**Time to call Emergency**	1122 (Pakistan) 999 (UK) 911 (USA)

ROSIER ASSESSMENT CHART

Date:_____ Time: _____

Symptom onset Date: _____ Time: _____

GCS: E_____   M_____   V_____

BP:_____

Blood Glucose:_____ (If <3.5 mmol/L, treat urgently and reassess once blood glucose is normal).

A. Has there been loss of consciousness or syncope?	Yes = -1		No = 0	
B. Has there been seizure activity?	Yes = -1		No = 0	
C. Is there a NEW ACUTE onset or on awakening from sleep?				
1. Asymmetric facial weakness	Yes = +1		No = 0	
2. Asymmetric arm weakness	Yes = +1		No = 0	
3. Asymmetric leg weakness	Yes = +1		No = 0	
4. Speech disturbance	Yes = +1		No = 0	

5. Visual field defect	Yes = +1		No = 0	
Total Score (-2 to +5)				

If total score is ≤0, stroke is unlikely but not completely excluded.

INVESTIGATIONS

- **CT/MRI of the brain:** To determine the pathology (ischemic or hemorrhagic), further delineate and localize the site of lesion in difficult/uncertain cases especially with MRI.

NCCT may show hyperdense vessel or dot sign suggestive of a thrombus.

- **CTA or MRA head & Neck:** To assess intra and extra-cranial vasculature. Most of the time, CTA head & neck are sufficient but in difficult and uncertain cases, MRA would be of help.

- **Carotid doppler:** To assess the extracranial internal carotid arteries (suitable patient for carotid endartrectomy).

- **CXR:** Any neoplasm, heart size.
- **ECG:** Arrythmias like AF, acute MI.
- **Echocardiography:** LV or atrial thrombus, PFO, Infective endocarditis, left atrial myxoma, papillary fibroelastoma
- **Lab studies:**

FBC: Polycythemia, thrombocytosis /thrombocytopenia, leukemia, Infection.

ESR /CRP /vasculitis screen: If CNS vasculitis /arteritis suspected.

Coagulation studies: May reveal coagulopathy. (If no clinical suspicion or known hematological disorder, thrombolysis should be performed without waiting for the results of hematologic tests).

Lipid profile, HbA1c

Basic chemistry panel: May reveal a stroke mimic (hypoglycemia, hyperglycemia, hyponatremia) or provide evidence of concurrent illness (DM, renal insufficiency).

Cardiac biomarkers: Association of CVD and CHD.

Toxicology screen: May identify intoxicated patient with behavior mimicking stroke or the use of sympathomimetics which can cause hemorrhagic or ischemic stroke.

Pregnancy test: For women of childbearing age; t-PA is relatively contraindicated in pregnancy.

STROKE MIMICS

Stroke mimic is defined as a manifestation of non-vascular disease process producing a stroke-like clinical picture.

The frequency of stroke mimics can be between 20% to 50% depending on the setting.

Though these mimics have characteristic features but sometimes in emergency, it could be challenging to differentiate these from the true stroke.

Early identification of stroke mimics could save the unnecessary investigations and lead to appropriate treatment.

MRI of the head is useful in acute setting in the challenging and uncertain cases to differentiate between the acute stroke and mimics.

Commonly encountered stroke mimics:

- Peripheral vertigo
- Migraine including hemiplegic variant
- Seizures /Todd's paralysis
- Functional symptoms
- SOL
- Sepsis in the background of previous stroke
- Multiple sclerosis
- Transient global amnesia (TGA)
- Hypo & Hyperglycemia
- Encephalitis
- Posterior reversible leukoencephalopathy synd

(PRES)
- Electrolytes imbalance
- Alcohol intoxication
- Side-effects of certain medications
- Focal neuropathies

CLASSIFICATION OF STROKE

◆ BAMFORD CLASSIFICATION

This is based on history and neurological examination.

TACS - Total Anterior Circulation Stroke:

All three of the following features:

a. Unilateral weakness &/or sensory deficit of face, arm and leg.

b. Homonymous hemianopia.

c. Higher cortical dysfunction (dysphasia, visuospatial neglect).

PACS - Partial Anterior Circulation Stroke: Any two of the above.

POCS - Posterior Circulation Stroke: One of the following features:

- Crossed signs: Ipsilateral cranial nerve palsy and contralateral motor/sensory deficit.
- Cerebellar dysfunction (e.g. nystagmus, ataxia).
- Conjugate eye movement disorder (e.g. horizontal gaze palsy, INO).
- Isolated homonymous hemianopia.
- Bilateral motor/sensory deficit.

LACS - Lacunar stroke: This is due to small vessel disease and there is no higher cortical dysfunction.

The common clinically encountered LACS are as follows:

- Pure motor stroke
- Pure sensory stroke
- Mixed sensory and motor stroke
- Ataxic hemiparesis
- Dysarthria-clumsy hand syndrome

◆ TOAST CLASSIFICATION

A systematic categorization of subtypes of ische-mic stroke mainly based on etiology supported by the ancillary diagnostic studies. Developed for the Trial of Org 10172 in Acute Stroke Treatment (TOAST).

There are five subtypes of ischemic stroke:

1. Large-artery atherosclerosis

2. Cardio-embolism

3. Small-vessel disease

4. Stroke of other determined etiology

5. Stroke of undetermined etiology

◆ NIH STROKE SCALE (NIHSS)

This 11-item scale measures the neurological deficit with 0-42 score. The higher score means deficit and probable poorer prognosis.

It is used worldwide as gold-standard scale in the clinical practice and clinical trials. It is rapid, reliable, and accurate, and can be performed by a broad-spectrum of healthcare providers.

NIHSS is what the patient is able to do, not what you think the patient can do.

If bedside NIHSS is 0, sit, stand and walk the patient (if safe) to check for the truncal, axial and gait ataxia.

NIH STROKE SCALE

Items	Scale definition Date/time----------	Score
1a. LOC	0 = Alert keenly responsive 1 = Not Alert but arousable by minor stimulation to obey, answer, respond 2 = Not Alert; requires repeat stimulation, obtunded, requires strong stimuli 3 = Reflex motor or autonomic effects response, totally unresponsive, flaccid	
1b. LOC Questions Ask the patient, the month & age.	0 = Answers both questions correctly 1 = Answers one question correctly 2 = Answers neither question correctly	
1c. LOC Commands Ask to open & close eyes, then grip & release with non-paretic hand.	0 = Performs both tasks correctly 1 = Performs one task correctly 2 = Performs neither task correctly	
2. Best Gaze Asked to	0= Normal 1= Partial gaze palsy; gaze is abnormal in one or both	

follow with eyes thru horizontal plane (or oculocephalic maneuver).	eyes but forced deviation or total gaze paresis is not present. 2 = Forced deviation; total gaze paresis not overcome by oculocephalic maneuver.	
3. Visual fields Tested with finger counting or visual threat (done by confrontation.	0 = No visual loss 1 = Partial hemianopia 2 = Complete hemianopia 3 = Bilateral hemianopia (including cortical blindness).	
4. Facial Palsy Asked to show teeth & raise eyebrows.	0 = Normal symmetrical movement 1 = Minor paralysis (flattened nasolabial fold, asymmetry on smiling) 2 = Partial paralysis (total or near total paralysis of lower face) 3 = Complete paralysis of one or both sides (no upper/lower face mvmt).	
5. Motor Arm Asked to extend	0 = No drift; limb holds 90º (or 45º) for full 10 seconds 1 = Drift; limb holds 90º (or 45º) but drifts down before	Left: Right:

arms (palm down) 90^0 (if sitting) or 45^0 (if supine) & hold for 10 seconds (count to 10). Begin with non-paretic limb.	full 10 seconds but does not hit bed or other support 2 = Some effort against gravity, limb cannot get to or maintain (if cued 90º or 45º) and falls to bed before 10 sec. 3 = Unable to overcome gravity; arm falls to bed immediately, minimum proximal movement present. 4 = No movement at all. UN (untestable) = Amputation, joint fusion: Explain---------	
6. Motor Leg While supine, asked to hold leg at 30^0 for 5 seconds (count to 5). Begin with non-paretic leg.	0 = No drift; leg holds 30º for full 5 seconds 1 = Drift, leg falls but does not hit bed 2 = Some effort against gravity, falls to bed w/in 5 sec 3 = Unable to overcome gravity; leg falls to bed immediately, minimum proximal movement present. 4 = No movement at all. UN = Amputation, joint fusion: Explain---------	Left: Right:
7. Limb Ataxia Finger-	0 = Absent 1 = Present in one limb 2 = Present in two limbs	

nose & heel-shin test on both sides.	UN = Amputation, joint fusion: Explain-----------	
8. Sensory Sensation or grimace to pin prick or withdrawal from noxious stimuli to limbs in obtunded or aphasic patient.	0 = Normal, no sensory loss 1 = Mild/moderate sensory loss; may be dulled/" Not as sharp" 2 = Severe/total sensory loss; not aware of face/arm/leg being touched	
9. Best Language	0 = No aphasia, normal 1 = Mild / moderate aphasia; some loss of fluency / comprehension, without limitation of expression of ideas. (can identify what is happening in picture) 2 = Severe aphasia; (cannot identify pictures) 3 = Mute; global aphasia; no usable speech; or auditory comprehension	
10. Dysarthria	0 = Normal articulation 1 = Mild / Moderate; slurs some words; understood w/	

	some difficulty 2 = Severe, so slurred as to be unintelligible; mute/ anarthria UN = Intubated or another physical barrier. Explain ------	
11. Extinction & In-attention Look at visual (from #3) and double simultaneous tactile. Do both arms & legs	0 = No abnormality 1 = Visual, tactile, auditory, spatial or personal in-attention or extinction to bilateral stimulation in one sensory modality 2 = Profound hemi-inatten-tion or inattention to more than one modality; does not recognize own hand; orients to only one side of space	
Sign	Total score	

◆ MODIFIED RANKIN SCALE

Modified Rankin Scale (mRS) is used to measure the functional independence and gait stability pre and post-stroke at 3-months.

Patients with pre-stroke ≤2 score were considered for acute reperfusion therapies in stroke trials.

Post-stroke score 0-2 is considered good outcome.

MODIFIED RANKIN SCALE

Score	Description
0	No symptoms at all
1	No significant disability despite symptoms; able to carry out all usual duties and activities
2	Slight disability: unable to carry out all previous activities, but able to look after own affairs without assistance
3	Moderate disability: requiring some help, but able to walk without assistance
4	Moderately severe disability: unable to walk without assistance and unable to attend to own bodily needs without assistance
5	Severe disability; bedridden, incontinent and requiring constant nursing care and attention
6	Dead

MANAGEMENT

Many TIAs and mild strokes can be managed in the out-patient setting. However, most of the stroke patients are admitted.

ACUTE MANAGEMENT

- **ABC:** Stabilize the patient.
- **Assess for thrombolysis/MT:** CT head, CT Perfusion and CT angiogram or MRI Head, MR perfusion and MR angiogram.
- **Thrombolysis:** In ischemic stroke, t-PA within 4.5 hours of onset reduces the disability.
- **Thrombectomy:** If large vessel occlusion with penumbra.
- **BP control**
- **Anti-platelet therapy:** For ischemic stroke (rule-out hemorrhage on brain imaging)
- **Treatment of stoke mimics:** Hypoglycemia, Hyperglycemia, Hyponatremia, Seizures/Todd's palsy, Hemiplegic migraine, Functional weakness, SOL, sepsis.

LONG-TERM MANAGEMENT

- Identify, address and treat the risk factors.
- Anti-platelet therapy for TIA and ischemic stroke.
- Control of HT: Aim <130/80 mmHg.
- Control of DM: Aim for HbA1c <7 mmol/l.
- Lipid lowering drugs: Aim for TC and LDL <3.8 and 1.8 mmol/l respectively. If diabetes or recurrent ischemic stroke, aiming for LDL <1.5 mm/l.
- Smoking cessation: Counselling, nicotine patches.
- Rehabilitation: Physiotherapy, and speech therapy.
- Occupational therapy: Various aids and modifica-

tions at home, e.g. stair railings, portable lavatories, bath rails, hoists, wheelchairs, tripods, modifications of doorways, sleep arrangements, stair lifts and kitchen modifications.

· Provision of "Meals on wheels" and "Get-up & Tuck-up" facilities.

OTHER CONSIDERATIONS

Surgical approaches:

- Carotid endarterectomy: TIA, minor strokes

- Hemicraniectomy: Malignant MCA syndrome

- Evacuation of hematoma: Impending herniation

- External ventricular drainage: Hydrocephalus

Dedicated stroke unit:

Patient care in dedicated stroke units has shown decreased rate of complications, early and safe discharges, patient, family and carers' satisfaction.

However, it has also shown reduction in the death and/or dependency at one year and need for institutional care.

Multidisciplinary approach:

Pathways are required for timely co-ordination to achieve best possible care and patient outcome among Emergency, General Medicine, Stroke Neurology, Neuroradiology, Neurosurgery, Intensive Care and Rehabilitation teams. In the long run, liaison among hospital, primary care physician, therapy team and Social workers is valuable.

Tele-stroke centers:

Experts in stroke care remotely assess a patient and consider thrombolysis (Drip n Ship model) and determine whether an immediate transfer to the tertiary care hospital is warranted in case of suspected large vessel occlusion and possible thrombectomy or more complex care needed.

Mobile Stroke Unit:

Many cities, in various countries, are now providing mobile stroke services (stroke ambulance) to reach the far-flung areas to assess and thrombolyse the eligible patients as soon as possible, as "time is brain", to reduce the disability.

POST-STROKE COMPLICATIONS

- **Infections (Pneumonia/UTI):** Pneumonia is the most common cause of morbidity and mortality in stroke patients. Dysphagia can lead to aspiration of both solids and liquids. Oral secretions as well as poor respiratory tract secretion-clearance could lead to pneumonia. Proper swallowing assessment with strict oral hygiene using oral cleansing and regular mouth-washes could prevent this devastating complication. Avoid unnecessary urinary catheterization. Early and prompt treatment of infections
- **Venous thrombo-embolism:** Good hydration, aspirin in ischemic stroke, and early mobilization. Intermittent pneumatic compression is preferable over prophylactic LMWH in immobile patients.
- **Bladder and bowel problems:**

Incontinence of bowel and bladder could be either due to immobilization as the patient can't go to the toilet /remove clothes or due to loss of awareness. Patient can develop urinary retention and constipation. Good toileting regimen, incontinence pads /condom catheters for dribbling /urinary catheterization for retention /laxatives and involvement of continence services.

- **Shoulder pain:** Common complications due to subluxation /dislocation /tendinitis /rotator-cuff injury. Proper positioning, including support of the joint with orthotics, as well as early occupational and/or physical therapy intervention with an analgesia. Pulling and pushing over paretic limb should be strongly discouraged.

- **Spasticity:** This could hamper the patient recovery. Physiotherapy, anti-spasticity medications (Baclofen and Tizanidine) and Botox injection in appropriately selected patients.
- **Seizures:** Most common with hemorrhagic stroke, anti-epileptics for seizures control. Primary prophylaxis with anti-epileptics is not recommended.
- **Pressure sores:** Pressure sores are common if the patient is left on hard surface or in one position for long time. Good nursing care, frequent position changing and avoiding hard surfaces.
- **Contractures:** Shortening of the soft-tissue structures spanning one or more joints could lead to contractures. Physiotherapy and splints.
- **Anxiety and depression:** Common among stroke survivors. Early screening with neuro-psychology input and anti-depressants as appropriate.
- **Falls and accidents:** Hemiparesis, sensory and visual impairment, gait imbalance and lack of confidence could lead to frequent falls, fractures and head injuries. Physiotherapy, occupational therapy and home appliances adjustment.

PROGNOSIS

Stroke is the 3rd common cause of death (mortality 11%). Early mortality is lesser for ischemic than for hemorrhagic stroke.

Poor outcome is more likely if there is coma, defect in conjugate gaze or severe hemiplegia.

Recurrence of stroke is common (10% in the first year).

Gradual improvement usually follows although patient may be left with severe residual disability. Of those who survive, about 1/3 return to independent mobility and 1/3 have severe disability requiring permanent institutional care. If sufficient language intelligible at 3 weeks, the outlook for fluent speech is good. However, many stroke patients are left with word-finding difficulties.

PROPHYLAXIS

Primary:
- Control of risk factors in the general population. Play grounds, parks, promotion of sports, anti-smoking and alcohol campaigns, checks on foods to avoid obesity, less salt and use of vegetable oil.
- Treatment of the predisposing conditions like DM, HT, AF and dyslipidemia.
- Prophylactic low-dose aspirin is not recommended as the risk of hemorrhage outweighs any benefit.

There is no role of carotid endarterectomy in asymptomatic carotid artery stenosis.

Postmenopausal HRT has shown no benefit.

Secondary:

- Lifestyle interventions: Smoking cessation, weight reduction, regular exercise and dietary modifications.
- Antiplatelets: Aspirin 75 mg is commonly used but Clopidogrel 75 mg OD is preferable over aspirin, as has modestly increased benefit in stroke prevention and decreased risk of GI and intracranial hemorrhage.
- Control of DM and HT.
- Lipid lowering drugs.
- Anticoagulants in selected patients.
- Carotid endarterectomy: Anterior circulation TIA and minor ischemic stroke with 70-99% symptomatic stenosis in women and 50-99% in men in the proximal ICA, provided the patient is neurologically and hemodynamically stable with life expectancy >3-5 years. It should be performed within 2 weeks of index event, with chances of perioperative complications and mortality <6%.

Carotid artery stenosis (NASCET criteria) needs to be confirmed by two modalities (Carotid doppler, CTA or MRA).

For total or near total occlusion, there is no role of carotid endarterectomy.

ISCHEMIC STROKE

I schemic stroke or "brain attack" is commonly caused by small vessel disease and thrombo-embolism. The clinical picture depends upon the site and extent of infarct. The site of infarct e.g. cortex, internal capsule or brainstem may be inferred from the pattern of physical signs.

Silent infarcts could be sometimes found on routine CT/ MRI head and treatment involves aggressive risk factors management. People with TIA may show infarcts on the brain imaging.

CLINICAL FEATURES

Most strokes are lacunar and mainly due to small vessel disease. The clinical signs depending upon the site and extent of lesion.

Hemiplegia/Hemiparesis: UMN lesion signs i.e. hypertonia, hyper-reflexia and extensor plantar response (Positive Babinski sign).

UMN Facial nerve palsy.

Dysphasia: When dominant hemisphere is involved.

Dysphagia, inattention, hemianopia.

Dysarthria, diplopia, ataxia, ipsilateral cranial nerve palsy.

Nystagmus, horizontal gaze palsy, internuclear ophthalmoplegia.

Weakness is maximal initially and recovers over days, weeks or months.

The affected limbs may at times be flaccid and areflexic initially (neuronal shock); hyper-reflexia occurs after a variable period.

INVESTIGATIONS

Brain imaging:

Patients suitable for acute reperfusion therapy (Thrombolysis /MT):

- NCCT, CTP and CTA (from arch of aorta to circle of Willis).
- MRI is increasingly being used in the diagnosis and management of acute ischemic stroke and is sensitive and relatively specific in detecting changes. It has some limitations, such as high cost, lack of wider availability and expertise, long scanning duration and contra-indications.
- DSA is not commonly used as it is invasive procedure and easy availability of CTA/MRA in detecting reliably high-grade stenosis and large vessel occlusion.

Patients not for acute reperfusion therapy:

NCCT followed by carotid doppler.
Antiplatelets

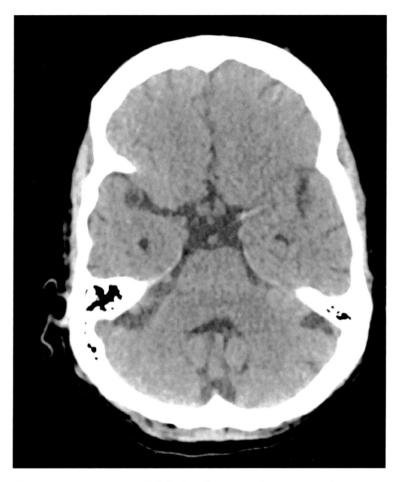

Figure: A 65-year-old lady, known hypertensive, presented with dense right hemiplegia, homonymous hemianopia and inattention. Non-contrast CT shows hyperdense left MCA - M1 sign suggestive of left MCA thrombus /occlusion.

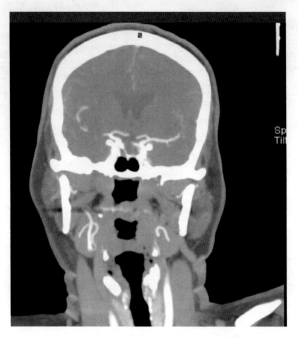

Figure: A 58-year old lady, known diabetic and hypertensive, presented with left hemiplegia, homonymous
hemianopia and neglect. Non-contrast CT Head was
normal. CT angiogram coronal view shows that right
MCA - M1 is occluded.

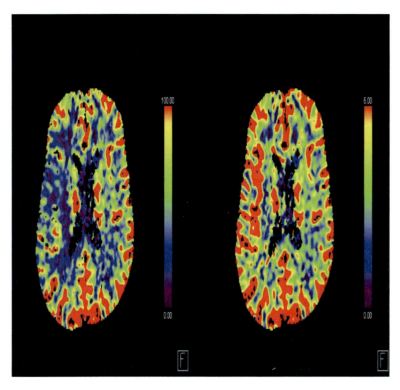

Figure: CT perfusion scan shows reduced cerebral blood flow in one and normal in other (mismatched perfusion defect) in the right MCA territory (penumbra - salvageable tissue).

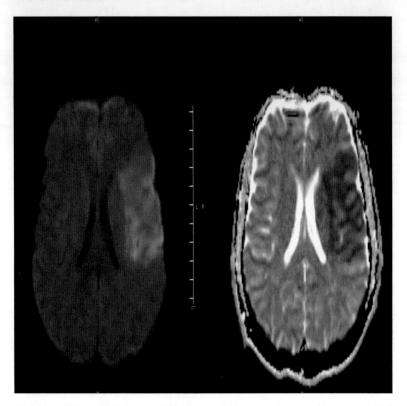

Figure: A 59 years, right-handed gentleman presented with right hemiparesis and dysphasia. MRI head shows areas of diffusion restriction as DWI bright, and ADC map dark - in keeping with left middle cerebral artery acute infarction.

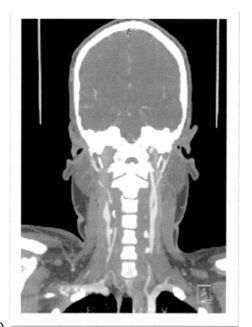

(a)

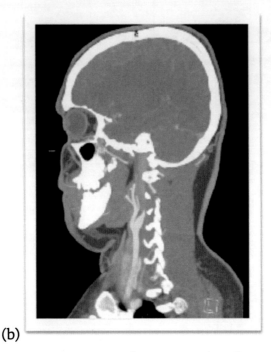

(b)

Figure: A young man of 26, previously well and fit, woke-up with headache, slurred speech, left-sided weakness and left visual inattention. CT angiogram coronal section showing tapering of right ICA and occlusion, while sagittal section showing tapering of right ICA – occluded suggestive of dissection.

Cardiac investigations:

ECG and Cardiac biomarkers: Association of CVD and CAD.

Echocardiography /24 hours Holter monitoring: To rule out cardiac pathology and paroxysmal AF, especially in cortical strokes. Sub-cortical lacunar stroke does not need cardiac investigations provided there is no other indication.

Other investigations:

Capillary Blood Glucose (Point of care): To rule out hypoglycemia as stroke mimic (usually ≤2.7 mmol/l (50 mg/dl) will cause neuroglycopenic symptoms.

FBC: May reveal a cause (polycythemia, thrombocytosis, thrombocytopenia, leukemia), and provide evidence of concurrent illness. If no previous history or clinical suspicion of hematological disorders, thrombolysis should be performed without waiting for FBC result.

Basic chemistry panel: May reveal a stroke mimic (hypoglycemia, hyperglycemia, hyponatremia) or provide evidence of concurrent illness (DM, renal insufficiency)

Coagulation studies: May reveal underlying coagulopathy - useful when fibrinolytics or anticoagulants are to be used.

Toxicology screen: To rule out intoxication mimicking stroke or the use of sympathomimetics, which can cause hemorrhagic or ischemic strokes.

Urine pregnancy test: For women of childbearing age; t-PA is relatively contra-indicated in pregnancy. Thrombolysis is a reasonable option in pregnancy for moderate to severe disabling stroke where anticipated benefit outweighs the risk of uterine bleeding.

MANAGEMENT
- **ABC**
- **Thrombolysis:**

Patients with disabling stroke, pre-stroke good baseline and no contraindications for thrombolysis, are given rt-PA (Alteplase - FDA approved) within 4.5 hours of onset or last well-known or at baseline state to reduce the disability.

It is critical not to delay thrombolysis after initial assessment and neuroimaging. Rest of the tests could be individualized except blood glucose (bedside) must precede thrombolysis.

NIH Stroke Scale (0-42 points) is used worldwide to assess the neurological deficit pre and post thrombolysis at 2 hrs, 24 hrs, day 7-10 or at discharge (whichever is earlier) and day-90.

- **Mechanical thrombectomy:**

If there is large vessel occlusion on CTA /MRA and large penumbra on CTP/MRP scan (salvageable tissue), MT is highly recommended.

MT as alternative to t-PA is under investigation.

The benchmarks for evaluation time of a patient for thrombolysis as suggested by NINDS and ACLS trials are given below.

BP targets:

For patients not for thrombolysis /MT but have acute severe co-morbidities (ACS, acute heart failure, aortic dissection, pre-eclampsia /eclampsia) the BP management should be individualized while maintaining good cerebral perfusion pressure. In general, 15% BP reduction is a reasonable option.

EVALUATION TIME FOR POTENTIAL THROMBOLYSIS CANDIDATE

Time Interval	Time Target
Door to doctor	10 min
Access to neurologic expertise	15 min
CT scan completion	25 min
CT scan interpretation	45 min
Door to treatment (thrombolysis)	60 min
Admission to stroke unit or ICU	3 hours

For thrombolysis/MT the BP <180/105 is maintained for at least next 24 hours.

BP <220/120 mmHg in patient who did receive t-PA/MT and have no acute severe co-morbidities, starting treatment within the first 48-72 hrs is not effective to prevent death or dependency.

BP ≥220/120 mmHg and patient not for t-PA/MT and no acute severe co-morbidities, the benefit of lowering BP in the first 48-72 hrs is uncertain. It is reasonable to reduce it by 15% in the first 24 hrs.

- **Anti-platelet therapy:** No anti-platelets for 24 hrs after t-PA. CT head is performed 24 hrs post t-PA to rule out bleed; if not, start anti-platelets.

Aspirin 300 mg PO STAT followed by 75-150 mg daily. Addition of clopidogrel could be considered for short duration on individual basis.

- **Swallowing assessment:** If fails to swallow, insert NG tube.
- **Oral hygiene:** Strict oral hygiene to reduce the risk of aspiration pneumonia – Regular oral cleansing /toileting/suctioning depending upon the oral secretions. Chlorohexidine oral mouth washes 4-6 hourly.
- **Venous thromboembolism prophylaxis:** Good hydration, Aspirin, early mobilization and intermittent pneumatic compression
- **Avoid urinary catheterization:** Unless retention; a source of infection.
- **Treatment of comorbid conditions:**

- HT

- Dyslipidemia

- Correct hypoxia if SaO_2 <94%. (For COPD patients the threshold is 88-92%).

- Correct hypo/hyperglycemia, Electrolyte imbalance:

Maintain Blood glucose at 6-11 mmol/l.

- Correct hypotension /Hypovolemia: 0.9% NaCl.

- Manage arrhythmias.

- Manage myocardial ischemia.

Life-style interventions: Smoking cessation /substance misuse avoidance, weight reduction, diet, regular exercise.

ROLE OF ANTIPLATELETS, ANTICOAGULANTS & THROMBOLYTICS IN ISCHEMIC STROKE

Antiplatelets:

Dispersible aspirin (75-300mg) is commonly used in the initial management of ischemic stroke.

If swallowing is an issue, aspirin 300 mg/day per rectum could be given.

In many RCTs (like International Stroke Trial, Chinese Acute Stroke Trial) its benefit and superiority over anticoagulants has been established.

Anticoagulants:

Anticoagulation has significant role in AF, LV thrombus and moderately severe mitral stenosis.

In Cardioembolic stroke due to AF, oral anticoagulation is usually started after 2 weeks of onset.

We have Vitamin K antagonist (warfarin) and NOACs (Rivaroxaban, Apixaban, dabigatran, Edoxaban). NOACs are better in NVAF than warfarin.

Currently, in vAF (Mechanical heart valves and mitral stenosis), warfarin in the only option.

Thrombolysis:

It has an established role in the early management of ischemic stroke. It reverts the thrombosed /obstructed vessel back to patency.

Its benefit outweighs the risk if given within 4½ hours of onset of symptoms. After that time the risk of hemorrhage surpasses the benefit and is not given.

Dose of t-PA (Alteplase): 0.9 mg/kg (max dose 90 mg), 10% is given in 1-2 minutes, and 90% over an hour as infusion.

Main side effects: 6-7% symptomatic intracranial hemorrhage (ICH), 2% fatal ICH, 1% orolingual angioedema.

NONVAVULAR AF RELATED ISCHEMIC STROKE & ORAL ANTICOAGULATION

AF is a major risk factor, leading to 4-5 times increased risk of ischemic stroke. These strokes are the most debilitating with higher mortality rate, longer inpatient stay and most likely needing institutionalized care. Patients with AF have a stroke risk of 4.5% per year, oral anticoagulation reduces it to 1.4% per year.

CHA_2DS_2-Vasc score is used to assess the future risk of ischemic stroke while HAS-BLED is used to predict future risk of bleeding due to anticoagulation.

Warfarin has been used for several decades. Time in therapeutic range (TTR) should be more than 70% to achieve satisfactory anticoagulation and protection in AF-related strokes. TTR is poorly achieved especially in Asian population.

NOACs have better efficacy and safety profile than warfarin. These have fewer drug interactions and there is no need for INR monitoring. It is important to prescribe correct dose of NOACs. Rivaroxaban should be taken with meals.

CHA$_2$DS$_2$-VASC SCORE

Risk factors	Score
CHF/LV dysfunction	1
Hypertension	1
Age≥75 years	2
Diabetes mellitus	1
Stroke/TIA/TE	2
Vascular disease (prior MI, PAD or aortic plaque)	1
Age 65-74 years	1
Sex category (female)	1
Total score	10

Key: TE – Thromboembolism, MI - Myocardial infarction, PAD – Peripheral arterial disease.

Maximum score is 10; score 0 in man and 1 in female does not warrant anticoagulation. For score 1 in men and 2 in female, consider oral anticoagulation. Score >1 in men and >2 in female, strong recommendation for oral anticoagulation.

HAS-BLED SCORE

Risk factors	Score
Hypertension	1
Abnormal renal and liver functions (1 point each)	1 or 2
Stroke	1
Bleeding	1
Labile INR (VKA)	1
Elderly (age >65 years)	1
Drugs and alcohol (1 point each)	1 or 2

Maximum score is 9. It has modifiable risk factors as well as sharing risk factors with CHA_2DS_2-Vasc score. HAS-BLED >3 predicts risk of bleeding and is not contraindication for oral anticoagulation but warrants caution and regular review of the patient.

COMPARISON OF COMMONLY USED NOACs

NOACs	Dabiga-tran	Apixa-ban	Rivaroxa-ban	Edoxa-ban
Action	Direct throm-bin inhibitor	Acti-vated factor Xa inhibitor	Activated factor Xa inhibitor	Acti-vated factor Xa inhibitor
Stand-ard dose	150 mg BID	5 mg BID	20 mg OD	60 mg OD
Dose in CKD	CrCl 30-49 ml/min, 110 mg BID	2 out-of 3: S. creatin-ine ≥1.5 mg/dl (≥133µ mol/l), age ≥80 years, weight ≤60 kg: 2.5 mg BID OR CrCl 15-29 ml/min or S. cre-atinine $^>$2.5mg/ dl (≥221 µmol/l): 2.5 mg BID	CrCl 15-49 ml/ min,15 mg OD	CrCl 15-49 ml/min, 30 mg OD
Not rec-om-mende	CrCl <30 mL/min	CrCl <15 mL/min	CrCl <15 mL/min	CrCl <15 mL/min

d

Key: CKD – Chronic kidney disease, CrCl – Creatinine clearance.

MECHANICAL THROMBECTOMY

M echanical thrombectomy (MT) is a well-established standard treatment for large vessel occlusion and salvageable tissue (large penumbra on CTP/MRP) in acute ischemic stroke in many countries.

Successful MT has shown significant improvement in patient's neurological status at 90 days and beyond.

Patients who are eligible for MT but are within the window for thrombolysis, should be given t-PA followed by MT. MT as alternative to t-PA is under investigation.

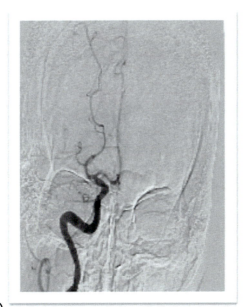

(a)

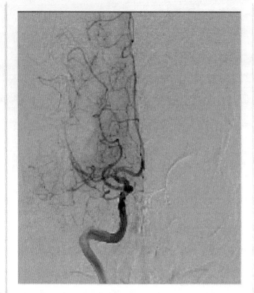

(b)

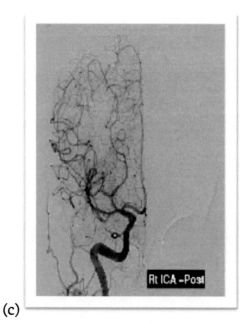

(c)

Figure: Mechanical thrombectomy; Digital subtraction angiogram (a) is showing right MCA-M1 occluded, (b) micro-catheter in M1 through right internal carotid artery, (c) opened right M1 - post-MT.

TRANSIENT ISCHEMIC ATTACK (TIA)

S udden-onset, focal neurological deficit due to vascular event in the brain that clears completely within 24 hours.

Most of the TIA symptoms last for seconds to minutes and the majority of patients are symptom-free in less than an hour.

TIA is a warning for major stroke; these patients have a 10% risk of getting stroke within 30 days, and half of these occur within 48 hours.

CINICAL FEATURES

Depend upon the site of lesion.

ANTERIOR CIRCULATION

(Carotid artery territory)

Can present as:

Amaurosis fugax

Hemiparesis, Hemianopia, Dysphasia

Hemi-sensory loss

POSTERIOR CIRCULATION

(Vertebrobasilar artery territory)

Can present as: Vertigo, diplopia, nausea/vomiting, ataxia, nystagmus, dysarthria, hemiparesis, visual field defects, hemisensory loss, amnesia, unconsciousness.

AMAUROSIS FUGAX

Transient monocular blindness due to retinal ischemia. It is due to small platelet emboli from an atherosclerotic lesion at the origin of internal carotid artery, causing transient occlusion of ophthalmic artery.

Patient may complain that vision was blurred in one eye or a shade swept up, down or across the field of vision or may say that the periphery of vision fades away.

INVESTIGATIONS

- CT Head and CTA or MRI of brain and MRA head and Neck
- Carotid doppler (for anterior circulation TIA) if CTA/MRA not available/inconclusive (for ICA).
- Blood glucose, HbA1c, FBC, U&Es, ESR /CRP/Lipid profile.
- CXR if indicated.
- ECG, Echocardiography and 24-48 hours Holter.

BRAIN-STEM STROKE

B rain-stem infarction causes complex patterns of dysfunction depending upon the site of lesion and its relation to the cranial nerve nuclei, long tracts and brain-stem connections.

It can present with:
- Crossed brain-stem syndromes
- Lateral, Medial, or Total Medullary syndrome
- Locked-in syndrome
- Comatose (Acute basilar artery occlusion, bilateral acute thalamic strokes)

CROSSED
BRAIN-STEM SYNDROMES

These syndromes are due to occlusion at different sites of vertebra-basilar circulation and thus lesions at different sites of the brainstem.

Weber syndrome: Ipsilateral III N palsy with contralateral hemiplegia. Site of lesion: Mid brain.

Benedikt syndrome: Ipsilateral III N palsy with contralateral involuntary movements (chorea). Site of lesion is mid brain with involvement of red nucleus.

Claude syndrome: III N palsy with contralateral ataxia.

Site of lesion is Red nucleus &/or dentate-rubro-thalamic tract. Due to occlusion of posterior cerebral artery at its origin.

Millard-Gubler syndrome: Ipsilateral VI and VII N palsy with contralateral Hemiplegia. Site of lesion: Pons.

Foville syndrome: Millard-Gubler syndrome (Hemiplegia + VI, VII N palsy) + Gaze palsy. As in Millard-Gubler syndrome, along with damage to supranuclear fibers controlling eye movements, so that lateral conjugate gaze towards the side of lesion may be paralyzed.

Raymong Cestan syndrome: Ipsilateral ataxia + coarse intention tremor + palsy of muscles of mastication and sensory loss on the face.

Contralateral loss of sensations in the body, hemiparesis of face & body and horizontal gaze palsy.

LATERAL MEDULLARY SYNDROME
(Wallenberg syndrome /PICA syndrome)

It results mainly from occlusion /dissection of either vertebral artery or posterior-inferior cerebellar artery (PICA).

CLINICAL FEATURES

Ipsilateral:

V N descending tract and nucleus: Pain, numbness, impaired sensation over half of face.

VI N: Diplopia, convergent squint.

Restiform body, cerebellar hemisphere, cerebellar fibers, spinocerebellar tract: Ataxia of limbs, falling to the side of lesion.

Vestibular nucleus: Nystagmus, diplopia, oscillopsia, vertigo, nausea, vomiting.

Descending sympathetic tract: Horner's syndrome (Partial ptosis, meiosis, anhidrosis).

IX, X N issuing fibers: Dysphagia, hoarseness, paralysis of palate, paralysis of vocal cord, diminished gag reflex.

Nucleus tractus solitarius: Loss of taste.

Cuneate and Gracile nucleus: Numbness of ipsilateral arm, trunk or leg.

Contralateral:

Spinothalamic tract: Impaired pain and thermal sensation over the contralateral half of the body, sometimes face.

MEDIAL MEDULLARY SYNDROME

It is due to occlusion of vertebral A, branch of vertebral A or lower basilar A.

CLINICAL FEATURES

Ipsilateral: XII N nucleus: Paralysis with atrophy of half of tongue.

Contralateral:

Pyramidal tract: Paralysis of arm and leg, sparing face.

Medial lemniscus: Impaired tactile and proprioceptive sense over half of body.

TOTAL MEDULLARY SYNDROME

Unilateral combination of Medial and Lateral Medullary syndromes.

It is due to occlusion of vertebral A.

LOCKED-IN SYNDROME

Interruption of descending and ascending long tracts in the brain stem, below the oculomotor nuclei, without disturbing consciousness.

As patient can't talk or move, it may be presumed that he can't understand, but this is not so.

Vertical eye movements and blinking are used to communicate in such patients.

HEMORRHAGIC STROKE

Hemorrhagic stroke can present as:

- Intra-cerebral or cerebellar hemorrhage
- Subarachnoid hemorrhage (SAH)
- Subdural or Extradural hematoma

Among stroke patients 15-20% are due to intracerebral or cerebellar hemorrhage.

It typically occurs in patients with HT. Rupture of micro-aneurysms (Charcot Bouchard nodes, 0.8-1 mm in diameter) is the principal cause.

It occurs at well-defined sites, like basal ganglia, thalamus, pons, cerebellum and subcortical white matter.

RISK FACTORS

- HT
- Thrombolytics and anticoagulants
- Bleeding disorders
- Cerebral aneurysms /AVM
- Cerebral amyloid angiopathy.

CLINICAL FEATURES

Sudden onset, rapidly progressive focal neurological deficit due to expanding hematoma in the brain.

Clinically there is no reliable way to distinguish intracerebral hemorrhage from infarct as both produce stroke.

Headache and coma favor intracerebral hemorrhage rather than infarct.

Pontine hemorrhage presents with high grade fever, quadriparesis, and constricted pupils.

INVESTIGATION

- **Non-contrast CT head:**

The diagnostic investigation. Hemorrhage is seen immediately in contrast to infarct. Because it is readily available, low cost, less time-consuming, it emains the investigation of choice to detect acute hemorrhage.

- **CT angiography:** When there is suspicion of ruptured AVM /aneurysm.
- **MRI head:** MRI with more modern sequencing as T2- weighted SWI and GRE is as sensitive as NCCT to detect acute hemorrhage. It can also detect old hemorrhages and chronic micro-hemorrhages as well.

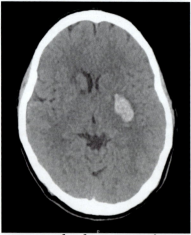

Figure: A 42-years male, hypertensive, non-compliant with medications, presented with right-sided weakness. Non-contrast CT brain is showing left basal ganglia hemorrhage secondary to hypertension

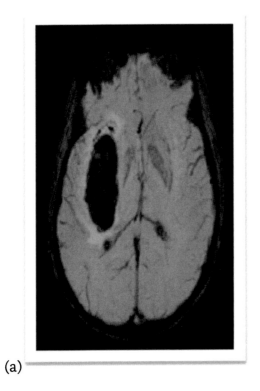

(a)

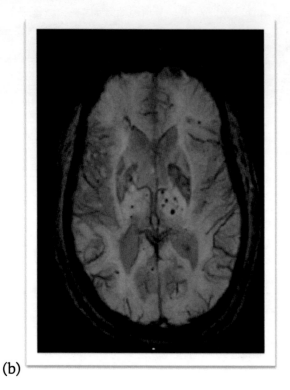

(b)

Figure: A 45 years gentleman, presented with dense left-sided weakness and low GCS. MRI-SWI (a) shows a large right basal ganglia hemorrhage, and (b) show multiple deep and superficial old micro-hemorrhages respectively.

MANAGEMENT

- ABC and general management as for infarct.
- Anti-platelets and anti-coagulants are contra-indicated.
- Reversal of INR.
- BP control: Aim for BP within 8 hours of onset between 130-150/80-90 mmHg, has shown modest functional benefit.
- Urgent neurosurgical intervention (hematoma evacuation, EVD) can be considered when intracerebral hematoma behaves as an expanding mass, causing deepening of coma, coning and hydrocephalus.

PROGNOSIS

Immediate prognosis of hemorrhage is worse than infarct; mortality is ~50%.

Once survived, the prognosis in terms of functional recovery is better than infarct.

SUBARACHNOID HEMORRHAGE

Spontaneous SAH is characterized by extravasation of blood into the subarachnoid space. It is a life-threatening neurosurgical emergency.

Its incidence is 6-20/100,000 population/year and comprises 2-5% of the CVA.

It is rare before the age of 20 and frequently occurs at 40-60 years age.

CLINICAL FEATURES

Headache: Sudden onset, thunderclap, worst ever head-ache, often occipital.

Nausea /vomiting.

Loss of consciousness: Remains comatose and drowsy for several hours to several days.

Signs of meningeal irritation: Neck stiffness, Kernig's sign.

Focal neurological deficits may occur.

There may be papilledema and sub-hyloid hemorrhage.

DIFFERENTIAL DIAGNOSIS

- Primary headaches (Migraine, cluster headache)
- Meningitis, encephalitis
- Reversible cerebral vasoconstriction syndrome
- Spontaneous ICH
- Temporal arteritis
- Arterial dissection (carotid /vertebral).
- Cavernous sinus thrombosis
- Pituitary apoplexy

CAUSES

- Cerebral aneurysms   85%
- No lesion found   10%
- AV malformation
- Other rare causes:

Bleeding disorders

Mycotic aneurysms

Vasculitis

Venous angiomas

Neoplasms

Sympathomimetic drugs

Extension of intra-cerebral hemorrhage into the sub-arachnoid space

RISK FACTORS

- Family history of SAH, African, Asian, Female sex, tobacco use
- Polycystic kidney disease
- Ehlers Danlos syndrome, Marfan's syndrome

Aneurysms at the Circle of Willis may cause symptoms either by spontaneous rupture or by the pressure on the surrounding structures, e.g. enlarging, unruptured posterior communicating artery aneurysm may cause painful III N palsy.

INVESTIGATIONS

- NCCT brain: Multi-model CT head has high sensitivity in the first 12 hours to detect SAH.
- LP: If CT head is normal.

Xanthochromia after 12 hours of ictus. If done earlier than 10-12 hours, it could turn out falsely negative.

If xanthochromia, the patient needs DSA and further intervention as appropriate; for those generally fit for surgery i.e. age <65 years and not in coma.

CSF loses its sensitivity after 2 weeks of symptoms onset.

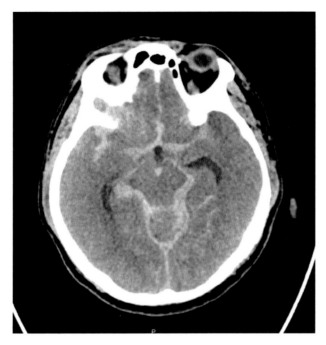

Figure: A 51 years old male was found unresponsive by friends. NCCT head shows diffuse SAH due to ruptured left posterior cerebral artery aneurysm, causing hydrocephalus as evidenced by dilated temporal horns of the lateral ventricles and blood in the sub-arachnoid space.

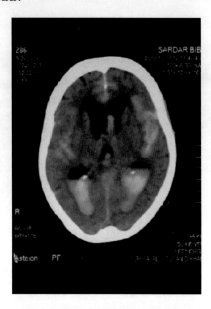

Figure: Non-contrast CT scan showing massive sub-arachnoid hemorrhage; blood is visible in both the Sylvian fissures and lateral ventricles as hyperdense shadows.

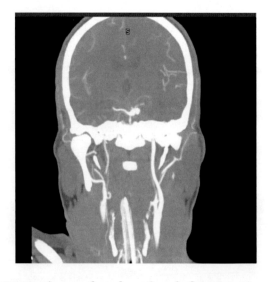

Figure: CT angiography showing left posterior cerebral

artery aneurysm.

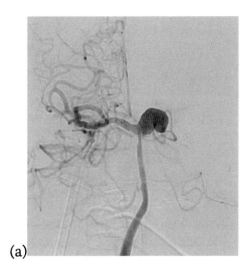

(a)

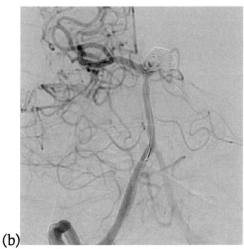

(b)

Figure: Digital subtraction angiography showing left posterior cerebral artery aneurysm (a) before and (b) after coiling.

MANAGEMENT

- Bed rest, hydration
- Elevate the head to 30^0
- Relieve the constipation
- Cough suppression
- Analgesia and Anti-emetics
- Control of HT
- Nimodipine: 60 mg 4 hourly for 21 days.
- Referral to specialist center for angiography and possible intervention.

Neurosurgical Management:

- Aneurysmal clipping /coiling/surgery.
- Micro-embolism and focal radiotherapy for AVM.

COMPLICATIONS

The causes of delayed neurological deficits in SAH.

Re-rupture: Mostly in 2-7 days.

Cerebral vasospasm: Leading to cerebral infarction 4-14 days after the onset in 30% patients.

Hydrocephalus

SUBDURAL HEMATOMA

A ccumulation of blood in the subdural space, following rupture of a vein. It is due to head injury (may be trivial), common in the elderly and alcoholics.

Headache, drowsiness and confusion are common. Symptoms often fluctuate.

Focal deficits such as hemiparesis or sensory loss may develop.

Epileptic fits occasionally occur.

Stupor and coma gradually ensue.

MANAGEMENT

Acute: Surgical evacuation.

Chronic: For old one corticosteroids and symptomatic therapy like anti-epileptics for fits.

EXTRADURAL HEMATOMA

E xtradural hematoma follows a linear skull vault fracture tearing a branch of middle meningeal artery resulting in rapid accumulation of blood in the extradural space.

It is almost always due to trauma.

Characteristically the patient presents with head injury, brief duration of unconsciousness followed by a lucid interval of recovery. Then progressive hemiparesis and stupor and rapid transtentorial coning, with first ipsilateral dilated pupil followed by bilateral fixed dilated pupils, tetraplegia and respiratory arrest.

MANAGEMENT

Immediate imaging: CT /MRI.

Urgent surgery: Neurosurgical intervention.

CEREBRAL VENOUS SINUS THROMBOSIS

C erebral venous thrombosis is a rare condition but could be potentially devastating. Early recognition and therapeutic intervention have decreased the morbidity and mortality.

Diagnosis is made on the basis of presentation and imaging studies while blood tests are done to delineate the underlying possible cause.

CLINICAL FEATURES

Headache (most common feature), nausea/vomiting, blurred vision, seizures, focal neurologic deficit, drowsiness /coma.

Extension of cavernous sinus thrombosis into the jugular bulb may cause jugular foramen syndrome due to compression.

RISK FACTORS

Dehydration, OCPs, HRT, ENT/CNS infections (meningitis, encephalitis, sinusitis), pregnancy/puerperium, head trauma and neurosurgical procedures such as dural taps and infusions into the internal jugular vein, permanent hypercoagulable states, malignancies.

INVESTIGATIONS

FBC, U&Es, ESR/CRP, LFTs, coagulation screen, thrombophilia screen, homocysteine level, ANA, ANCA.

NCCT/MRI head, and CTV/MRV, fundoscopy for disc changes/papilledema.

Lumbar puncture if CNS infection suspected.

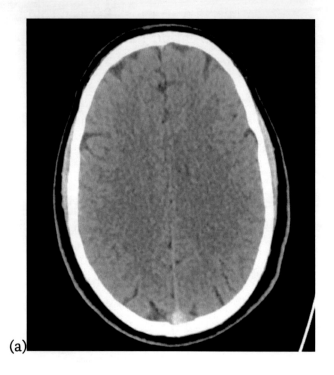

(a)

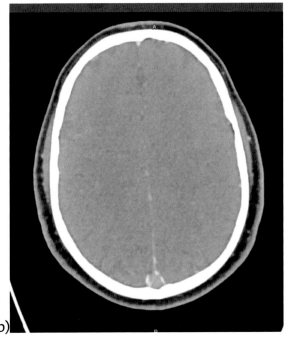

(b)

Figure: (a) Non-contrast CT head shows hyperdense sign and (b) CT Venogram shows empty delta sign suggestive of cerebral venous sinus thrombosis.

TREATMENT

◆ Stabilize the patient: ABC

◆ General medical management: Similar to arterial stroke with further consideration for the following:

◆ Correct the underlying dehydration.

◆ If signs of raised ICP (e.g. visual symptoms with papilledema), consider starting acetazolamide.

◆ Lumbar puncture is an option in carefully selected patients to relieve the pressure.

◆ Antiepileptics for seizures.

Septic CVST: Treat the underlying infection. Aggressive antibiotic therapy and neurosurgical/ENT opinion as appropriate. Role of anti-coagulation is not well established in septic CVST.

Non-septic CVST: Start LMWH (enoxaparin 1.5 mg/kg per day) followed by either warfarin or NOACs (Apixaban, Dabigatran, Rivaroxaban).

Provoked CVST: Oral anticoagulation for 3-6 months. CTV/MRV should be repeated after 3 months, if almost full recanalization, oral anticoagulation should be stopped.

Unprovoked CVST: Oral anticoagulation for 6-12 months . Consider repeat CTV/MRV near completion of oral anticoagulation course to assess for recanalization.

CVST during pregnancy: Full dose LMWH during pregnancy followed by either LMWH or VKA for ≥6 weeks postpartum (for a total minimum duration of therapy of 6 months).

Thrombophilia workup should be done at least 4-6 weeks post-delivery.

If there is underlying permanent hypercoagulable state, consider lifelong oral anticoagulation provided no contraindications.

Though hemorrhagic venus infarct /venus hemorrhage is not contraindication for anticoagulation in CVST, but careful neuro vital monitoring is essential as hematoma may expand and lead to suspension of anticoagulation.

Neurosurgical interventions:

Large intraparenchymal lesion causing herniation - consider hemicraniectomy. Drainage of subdural empyema/abscess.

LAND-MARK TRIALS

The initial two major trials of aspirin in acute ische-mic stroke, IST and CAST taken together, show reliably that aspirin started early produces a significant net benefit, with fewer deaths or non-fatal strokes in the first few weeks, and with fewer patients dead or de-pendent after some weeks or months of follow-up.

◆ IST

International Stroke Trial

This trial established the role of aspirin in decreasing the death and recurrent stroke and also the superiority of aspirin over heparin in the management of ischemic stroke.

In this RCT, 19,435 patients with acute ischemic stroke were randomized to heparin, aspirin or none.

The primary outcomes were death within 14 days and death or dependency at 6 months.

Among heparin-allocated patients, there were non-sig-nificant fewer deaths in 14 days.

Compared with 5000 IU BD heparin, 12,500 IU BD was associated with significantly more transfused or fatal extra-cranial bleeds, more hemorrhagic strokes, and more deaths or non-fatal strokes in 14 days. At 6 months the percentage of death or dependency was identical in both groups.

In aspirin-allocated patients there were non-significantly fewer deaths in 14 days. At 6 months there was non-significant trend towards a smaller percentage of dead or dependent; after adjustment for baseline prognosis the benefit was significant.

Aspirin-allocated patients had significantly fewer recurrent ischemic strokes in 14 days with no significant excess of hemorrhagic strokes, so the reduction in death or non-fatal recurrent stroke with aspirin was significant.

Ref: Lancet 1997; 349:1569-81.

◆ CAST
Chinese Acute Stroke Trial

> This trial established that aspirin decreased the death and recurrent stroke in patients with acute ischemic stroke.

In this RCT, 21,106 patients with acute ischemic stroke were randomized to get aspirin or placebo started within 48 hours of onset and continued in-hospital for up to 4 weeks.

At discharge, there were fewer deaths or dependency in favor of aspirin than placebo.

There were significantly fewer recurrent ischemic strokes in aspirin-allocated group but non-significantly more hemorrhagic strokes.

For the combined in-hospital endpoint of death or non-fatal stroke, there was a proportional risk reduction with aspirin.

Ref: Lancet 1997; 349:1641-9.

◆ NINDS
National Institute of Neurological Disorders and Stroke

> This study established that despite an increased incidence of symptomatic intracerebral hemorrhage, treatment with IV t-PA within 3 hours of onset of ischemic stroke improved the clinical outcome.

In this RCT, 624 patients with clinical diagnosis of ischemic stroke with measurable disabling neurologic deficit were given IV t-PA or placebo. The trial had two parts. Part 1 (291 patients) tested whether t-PA had clinical activity, as indicated by improvement of 4 points over base-line values in NIH stroke scale or resolution of neurologic deficit within 24 hours of onset of stroke. Part 2 (333 patients) used a global test statistic to assess clinical outcome at 3 months, according to Barthel index, modified Rankin scale, Glasgow outcome scale, and NIHSS.

In part 1, there was no significant difference between the two groups in the percentages of patients with neurologic improvement at 24 hrs, although a benefit was observed for t-PA at 3 months for all four outcome measures.

In part 2, the long-term clinical benefit of t-PA predicted by results of part 1 was confirmed. As compared with placebo, patients treated with t-PA were at least 30% more likely to have minimal or no disability at 3 months on assessment scales. Mortality at three months was 17% in t-PA and 21% in placebo group (p = 0.30).

Symptomatic intracerebral hemorrhage within 36 hrs after the onset of stroke occurred in 6.4% patients given t-PA but 0.6% in placebo (P<0.001).

Ref: N Engl J Med 1995; 333:1581-8.

◆ ECASS

European Cooperative Acute Stroke Study

> IV alteplase between 3 and 4.5 hours after symptoms improved outcomes in patients with acute ischemic stroke.

In this RCT, 623 patients in 14 European countries with acute ischemic stroke in whom IV t-PA could be initiated within 6 hrs from the onset of symptoms were evaluated by neurological examination and cerebral CT scans.

Treatment effect was evaluated using the Barthel Index and Modified Rankin Scale at 90 days. The clinical course was evaluated by repeated neurological ratings on Scandinavian Stroke Scale. Adverse events were evaluated by repeating CT scans at 24 h and at 7 days. Overall mortality was 18.9%. The incidence of cerebral bleeding complications associated with clinical deterioration was 6.5%.

Ref: Eur J Neurol 1995; 1:213-9.

◆ PROACT II
Prolyse in Acute Cerebral Thromboembolism II

> Treatment with IA pro-urokinase within 6 hours of onset of acute ischemic stroke caused by MCA occlusion significantly improved the clinical outcome at 90 days; despite an increased frequency of early symptomatic intracranial hemorrhage.

In this RCT, 180 patients with acute ischemic stroke of less than 6 hrs duration caused by angiographically proven occlusion of MCA were randomized to receive 9 mg of IA r-prourokinase plus heparin or heparin only.

The primary outcome was based on the proportion of patients with slight or no neurological disability at 90 days as defined by a modified Rankin score of 2 or less. Secondary outcomes included MCA recanalization, frequency of intracranial hemorrhage with neurological deterioration, and mortality.

For the primary analysis, 40% of pro-urokinase patients and 25% controls had a modified Rankin score of 2 or less (p=0.04). Mortality was 25% for pro-urokinase group and 27% for controls. Recanalization rate was 66% for the proUK group and 18% for control group (p<0.001).

Intracranial hemorrhage with neurological deterioration within 24 hrs occurred in 10% of pro-urokinase patients and 2% of controls (p=0 .06).

Ref: JAMA 1999; 282:2003-11.

◆ **EXTEND**

Thrombolysis guided by perfusion imaging up to 9 hours after onset of stroke

> Patients with ischemic stroke and salvageable brain tissue, alteplase between 4.5 and 9 hrs after stroke onset results in a higher percentage of patients with no or minor neurologic deficits. There were more cases of symptomatic cerebral hemorrhage in alteplase group than placebo.

In this RCT, 225 patients with ischemic stroke who had hypoperfused but salvageable regions of brain detected on automated perfusion imaging, were assigned to IV alteplase or placebo between 4.5 and 9 hours after the onset of stroke. The primary outcome was a score of 0 or 1 on modified Rankin scale, at 90 days.

The primary outcome occurred in 40 (35.4%) in alteplase group and in 33 (29.5%) in placebo group (adjusted risk ratio, 1.44; 95% CI, 1.01 to 2.06; P=0.04). Symptomatic intracerebral hemorrhage occurred in 7 patients (6.2%) in alteplase group and 1 patient (0.9%) in placebo group (adjusted risk ratio, 7.22; 95% CI, 0.97 to 53.5; P=0.05). A secondary ordinal analysis of the distribution of scores on the modified Rankin scale did not show a significant between-group difference in functional improvement at 90 days.

Ref: N Engl J Med 2019; 380:1795-1803.

◆ CAST

Stroke Prevention by Aggressive Reduction in Cholesterol Levels

> This study showed that statins reduced the incidence of strokes and cardiovascular events in patients with recent stroke or TIA and without known CAD.

In this study, 4731 patients with stroke or TIA 1-6 months before study, with LDL-C levels 100-190 mg/dL and no known coronary heart disease were assigned to double-blind treatment with 80 mg atorvastatin per day or placebo and followed-up for a median 4.9 years.

The mean LDL-C level during the trial was 73 mg/dL among patients receiving atorvastatin and 129 mg/dL among placebo group.

Patients receiving atorvastatin had a significant 5-year absolute reduction in risk of fatal or nonfatal stroke.

The five-year absolute reduction in risk of major CV events was significantly reduced in atorvastatin group.

The overall mortality rate was similar, as were the rates of serious adverse events. Elevated liver enzyme values were more common in patients taking atorvastatin.

Ref: N Engl J Med 2006; 355:549-59.

◆ NIMODIPINE Trial

Cerebral arterial spasm – a controlled trial of Nimodipine in patients with SAH

> This study showed that CCB, nimodipine decreased the risk of severe neurologic deficits due to cerebral arterial spasm in the 21 days after SAH.

In this RCT, 125 neurologically normal patients with intracranial aneurysms within 96 hours of SAH were randomized to determine whether treatment with nimodipine would prevent or reduce the severity of ischemic neurologic deficits from arterial spasm.

A deficit from cerebral arterial spasm that persisted and was severe or caused death by the end of 21-day treatment occurred in 8 of 60 patients given placebo and 1 of 56 given nimodipine (p=0.03).

Analysis of amount of basal subarachnoid blood on pre-entry CT scans in patients with deficits from spasm showed that an increase in subarachnoid blood was not associated with a worse neurologic outcome among patients who received nimodipine, unlike in patients given a placebo.

Ref: N Engl J Med 1983; 308:619-24.

CHRONIC OBSTRUCTIVE PULMONARY DISEASE

Patients with chronic obstructive pulmonary disease (COPD) are quite common and thus easily available as long-case for the exams.

SUMMARY

This gentleman, Mr. Bukhshi, 58 years old, from Rawlakote, Kashmir, is suffering from cough with expectoration for the last 16 years. The amount and color of sputum varies from time to time. At the moment it is about 2 TSF a day and yellow in color, without any blood. He recalls the history of hospitalization with increasing cough and SOB most of the winters. He is an ex-smoker for the last 5 years after >20 years of heavy smoking history. This time he presented with increasing SOB, cough, yellow expectoration and fever for 2 weeks.

On examination, he shows signs of heart failure i.e. pedal edema, and raised JVP, along with bilateral course rhonchi and scattered crackles which change their character with coughing.

He has got:

COPD with acute exacerbation and corpulmonale.

MANAGEMENT PLAN

I will monitor his vital signs including the SaO_2 (by pulse oximetry).

I will perform a chest x-ray to check for any sign of pneumonia or pneumothorax and for the heart size.

I will perform an ECG and echocardiography to check for signs of pulmonary HT and corpulmonale.

I will send his sputum samples for microscopy and culture, apart from the baseline investigations like FBC, blood sugar, U&Es, and urinalysis.

His acute condition is now settled down; I would have managed his acute condition by O_2 inhalation (24%) via nasal cannula, Bronchodilators by nebulization, Antibiotics according to the hospital antimicrobial policy preferably including a macroloid, and corticosteroids.

Before discharge, I will shift his nebs to inhalers (LABA /LAMA $\pm$ ICS) and parenteral medications to oral. I will also consider and assess him for LTOT.

Later, I will advise Influenza (flue jab), and Pneumococcal vaccination for the future.

After discharge from the hospital, he will need GP appointment after 2 weeks and Specialist appointment after 4-6 weeks-time. His GP may arrange for home visits by the community respiratory nurse if needed.

DISCUSSION

During discussion the following questions may be asked in one way or the other. Tips for properly answering these questions are given in the following sections:

➢ Criteria for the diagnosis of COPD.

➢ Precipitants of acute exacerbation of COPD.

➢ Management of patient with COPD exacerbation.

➢ Complications of COPD.

➢ Indications or criteria for LTOT in COPD.

➢ Hazards of smoking and how to stop smoking.

➢ E-Cigarettes; merits and demerits.

➢ Land-mark trials regarding management of COPD.

➢ Land-mark trials for prescribing LTOT.

CHRONIC OBSTRUCTIVE PULMONARY DISEASE

C hronic obstructive pulmonary disease is characterized by persistent respiratory symptoms and airflow limitation due to airway and/or alveolar abnormalities, usually caused by exposure to noxious particles or gases.

Smoking is the main risk factor but other environmental exposures and air pollution may also contribute.

Chronic bronchitis vs. Emphysema: COPD is a spectrum of these two processes - one of these usually predominates in a specific patient.

Chronic bronchitis is a clinical diagnosis characterized by cough with expectoration on most of the days for at least three consecutive months of two consecutive years.

Emphysema is a pathologic diagnosis characterized by destruction of alveolar walls.

In a rare case, bronchial asthma and COPD may overlap and the condition is then labeled as chronic airflow limitation.

The global prevalence of COPD is estimated to be 7% to 19% from various studies. The prevalence varies in different regions of the world. The Burden of Obstructive Lung Disease (BOLD) study found a global prevalence of 10.1%; 11.8% in men and 8.5% in women.

It is the 4th leading cause of death in the world.

CLINICAL FEATURES

Cough, expectoration and dyspnea are the frequent symptoms.

Certain features can differentiate between the patients with predominant chronic bronchitis or emphysema.

Patients with predominant chronic bronchitis (previously called blue-bloaters) are usually obese and typically have frequent cough and expectoration. Coarse rhonchi may be heard on auscultation. They may also show signs of corpulmonale such as edema and cyanosis.

While those with predominant emphysema (previously called pink-puffers) are usually thin, with barrel-shaped chest and typically have little or no cough or expectoration. They may assist their breathing by pursed lips. The chest may be hyper-resonant, with wheezing and the heart sounds may feel distant.

Exacerbation:

Acute worsening of respiratory symptoms.

The most common precipitant of acute exacerbation is infection. The others are environmental changes and pollution.

DIAGNOSIS

COPD is diagnosed on the basis of spirometry, which should be performed in patients with clinical features or risk factors for COPD.

Post–bronchodilator FEV1/FVC <0.7 is the spirometric criteria for airflow limitation.

Patients can then be evaluated for severity. Global Strategy for the Diagnosis, Management & Prevention of COPD (GOLD) guidelines categorize the patients by:

- Airflow limitation
- Symptoms /risk of exacerbation.

Dyspnea is defined according to the COPD Assessment Test (CAT) which is actually a modified MRC score for grading of dyspnea.

Younger patients (age <40) should also be screened for α-1 antitrypsin deficiency. Other investigations such as thoracic imaging, lung volume studies, diffusion capacity and oximetry may also be required.

MANAGEMENT
The goals of treatment are to;
- Stabilize the decline in lung function
- Reduce the rate of exacerbations
- Reduce the hospitalizations and mortality

- Manage the dyspnea
- Improve the exercise tolerance and quality of life

Non-pharmacologic:

- Smoking cessation and reduction of exposure to other pollutants.
- Influenza and pneumococcal vaccination.
- Pulmonary rehabilitation to improve the symptoms and Qol.
- LTOT in patients with severe resting hypoxemia.
- Interventional bronchoscopy or surgery (lung volume reduction or bullectomy) in selected cases.

Pharmacologic:

Bronchodilators and anti-inflammatory agents are the main stay of therapy.

- **β2-agonists:** Short-acting e.g. Salbutamol and long–acting: e.g. Salmeterol.
- **Anti-muscarinics:** Short-acting: e.g. Ipratropium and long-acting: e.g. Tiotropium.
- **Xanthine derivatives:** e.g. Theophylline.
- **Inhaled corticosteroids:** e.g. Beclomethasone.
- **Phosphodiesterase-4 inhibitors:** e.g. Roflumilast (reduces exacerbations and improves the lung function).
- **Azithromycin/erythromycin:** Reduce the exacerbations.
- **Oral corticosteroids:** e.g. Prednisone.

TREATMENT PRINCIPLES

According to the GOLD guidelines 2020:

Stable COPD:

Grade A: Short or long–acting bronchodilator.

Grade B: Initially LABA or LAMA. The two combined in case of persistent symptoms. Combinations improve the lung function, symptoms, and QoL, and are more effective than monotherapy in preventing AEs.

Combining two complementary agents with different mechanism of action reduces the risk of AEs as compared to increasing the dose of a single agent.

Grade C: Initially LAMA; if exacerbations occur, then LAMA/LABA combination (preferred) or LABA/ICS.

Grade D: Initially LABA/LAMA combination (preferred), LAMA as monotherapy, or LABA/ICS.

If there are still exacerbations, triple therapy LABA/LAMA/ICS or LABA/ICS with LAMA added later if necessary.

Phosphodiesterase-4 inhibitor can be added in patients with AEs despite treatment with LABA/ICS or LABA/LAMA/ICS.

Exacerbations:

Mild: SABA and/or SAMA.

Moderate: Short-acting bronchodilators plus antibiotics and/or oral corticosteroids.

Severe: Hospitalization and possible respiratory support.

COMPLICATIONS
- Acute exacerbation
- Pneumonia
- Pulmonary hypertension
- Respiratory failure
- Corpulmonale

COR PULMONALE

Pulmonary hypertension leading to right ventricular hypertrophy or failure, in a patient with chronic pulmonary or thoracic wall disorder.

On examination the patient has edema, tachycardia, raised JVP, and heart examination reveals RV heave and other signs of heart failure.

ECG shows tachycardia or AF, Right axis deviation, RA and RV enlargement.

Chest x-ray may reveal cardiomegaly.

MANAGEMENT

- Low salt diet.
- Fluid restriction: 1.5 L/day.
- Oxygen inhalation: Assess for LTOT.
- Diuretics: Loop diuretics (Furosemide).
- Anti-platelets.
- Monitor the renal function.

There is no evidence for the use of ACE-Is, CCBs, α-blockers, or digoxin in the management of corpulmonale.

LONG-TERM OXYGEN THERAPY

Long-term oxygen therapy (LTOT) is indicated in the management of COPD with severe hypoxemia.

It is also prescribed in certain other conditions like pulmonary fibrosis with respiratory failure.

In COPD, assessment for LTOT should be done when the patient is clinically stable.

- PaO_2 <7.3 kPa &/or PCO_2 >6 KPa on 2 occasions 3 wks apart.
- FEV1 <1.5 L with <15% improvement after bronchodilator.
- Carboxyhemoglobin <10% i.e. the patient is not smoking.

Oxygen should be given at least 15 hours a day using oxygen concentrator (1-4 L/min) through nasal prongs. Night time to be included as hypoxemia worsens during sleep.

LAND-MARK TRIALS

For patients with COPD, the fixed-dose inhaled LABA/LAMA combinations as baseline therapy has been shown to have better efficacy as compared to mono-therapy.

It is more beneficial as compared to LABA/ICS. In addition to efficacy, ICS treatment is associated with increased risk of pneumonia.

◆ LANTERN

This study supported the use of LABA/LAMA, as an alternative treatment, over LABA/ICS, in the management of moderate-to-severe COPD with a history of ≤1 exacerbation in previous year.

In this RCT, 744 patients with moderate-to-severe COPD with history of ≤1 exacerbations in the previous year were randomized to LABA/LAMA or LABA/ICS for 26 weeks.

LABA/LAMA demonstrated statistically significant superiority to LABA/ICS. It significantly reduced the rate of moderate or severe exacerbations over LABA/ICS.

Ref: Int J Chron Obstruct Pulmon Dis 2015; 10:1015-26.

◆ ILLUMINATE

> In moderate to severe COPD without history of AEs in the previous year, LABA/LAMA combination was significantly superior to LABA/ICS therapy.

In this RCT, 523 patients GOLD stages II–III, without exacerbations in the previous year were randomly assigned LABA/LAMA or LABA/ICS for 26 weeks.

LABA/LAMA combination was found significantly superior to LABA/ICS therapy.

Ref: Lancet Respir Med 2013; 1:51-60.

◆ FLAME

> LABA/LAMA was more effective than LABA/ICS in preventing COPD exacerbations in patients with a history of exacerbation during the previous year. The incidence of pneumonia was significantly lower in LABA/LAMA group.

In this RCT, 3362 patients of COPD with a history of at least one AE during the previous year were randomly assigned to LABA/LAMA or LABA/ICS for 52 weeks.

LABA/LAMA was more effective than LABA/ICS in reducing the annual rate of AEs. The incidence of pneumonia was significantly lower in LABA/LAMA group.

Ref: N Engl J Med 2016; 374:2222-34.

◆ WISDOM

In severe COPD receiving LABA/LAMA/ICS, the risk of AEs was similar among those who discontinued inhaled glucocorticoids. However, there was a greater decrease in lung function during the final step of glucocorticoid withdrawal.

In this RCT, 2485 patients with history of exacerbation of COPD received triple therapy LAMA/LABA/ICS for a 6-week run-in period. They were then randomly assigned to continue the triple therapy or withdraw ICS in three steps over a 12-week period.

At 12 months follow-up the risk of exacerbations was similar in both groups, although there was greater decrease in lung function during the final step of glucocorticoid withdrawal.

Ref: N Engl J Med 2014; 371:1285-94.

◆ INSTEAD

Patients with moderate COPD and no exacerbations in the previous year can be safely switched from LABA/

> ICS to LABA only.

In this RCT, 581 patients with moderate COPD and no exacerbations for a year before the study. They had been receiving LABA/ICS for ≥3 month. They were assigned to LABA or ICS.

There were no significant difference between treatments in terms of breathlessness or health status or exacerbation rates at weeks 12 or 26.

Ref: Eur Respir J 2014; 44:1548-56.

◆ OPTIMO

> Withdrawal of ICS, in COPD patients at low risk of exacerbation, can be safe provided that patients are left on maintenance treatment with long-acting bronchodilators.

In this study, 914 patients having COPD patients at low risk of exacerbation on bronchodilators and ICS. Their ICS was either continued or withdrawn.

After 6 months, there was no difference between the two groups in deterioration of lung function or exacerbation rate, suggesting that ICS was safe to withdraw in COPD patients at low risk of exacerbation if long-acting bronchodilator was maintained.

Ref: Respir Res 2014; 15:77.

TRIALS FOR LONG-TERM OXYGEN THERAPY

The benefits of LTOT in severely hypoxemic COPD patients were shown in trials in the early 1980. However, these benefits were not replicated in some later trials, even though a number of studies reported benefits in breathlessness. The issue of LTOT for patients with moderate hypoxemia, hypoxemia only during sleep and exercise-induced hypoxemia has remained controversial. Some of the studies did not show any survival benefit in patients with moderate hypoxemia.

◆ NOTT
Nocturnal Oxygen Therapy Trial

This study established the superiority of continuous oxygen therapy ($\geq$19 hours) over nocturnal oxygen ($\leq$13 hours) in patients with hypoxemic COPD.

In this study, 203 patients with hypoxemic COPD were randomly allocated either to nocturnal oxygen therapy (NOT) group $\leq$13 hrs, or to continuous oxygen therapy (COT) group $\geq$19 hrs/day and followed for 12 months.

The overall mortality in NOT group was significantly higher than COT group.

Ref: Respir Care 1981; 26:63-5.

◆ **MRC Trial**

Medical Research Council Oxygen therapy Trial

> This study established the benefit of LTOT in patients
> with COPD with chronic hypoxic corpulmonale.

In this RCT, 87 patients of COPD with severe hypoxemia,
CO_2 retention, and history of CCF were randomized to
oxygen therapy or no oxygen. Oxygen was given by
nasal prongs for at least 15 h daily, at 2 l/min and followed for 5 years.

Mortality was significantly less in oxygen treated patients as compared to controls. Physiological measurements suggested that oxygen did not slow the progress
of respiratory failure in those who died early. However,
in long term oxygen, oxygenation did seem to stop deterioration.

Ref: Lancet 1981; 1:681-6.

◆ **LOTT**

Long-Term Oxygen Treatment Trial

> This study showed that LTOT had no benefit in pa-
> tients with stable COPD and resting or exercise-in-

duced moderate hypoxemia.

In this study, 738 patients with stable COPD and resting or exercise-induced moderate hypoxemia were randomized to receive long-term supplemental oxygen or none and followed for 1 to 6 years. Those with resting hypoxemia were prescribed 24-hour oxygen, and those with exercise-induced hypoxemia during exercise and sleep.

LTOT had no survival benefit or benefit in terms of hospitalization or exacerbation rate.

Ref: N Engl J Med 2016; 375:1617-27.

CHRONIC KIDNEY DISEASE

SUMMARY

This gentleman, Mr. Khan from Peshawar, age 45 years presented to A&E with SOB, nausea, vomiting, malaise, body aches and swelling of his feet for the last 10 days.

He is a known patient of T2D and HT for more than 10 years. He has a poor compliance to treatment and dietary restrictions.

On examination: His pulse is 72 beats/min, regular, BP 140/88 mmHg on medications (Amlodipine 5 mg + Losartan 50 mg) and has got mild pedal edema.

Cardiovascular examination revealed a pericardial rub and his chest has scattered crackles in both the lower zones.

He has got:

Type 2 diabetes, HT and CKD with Pericarditis.

MANAGEMENT PLAN

I will perform RFTs (MSU with microscopy, C/S if required, U&Es, Creatinine, eGFR), Serum proteins, and USG for kidneys, ureters, bladder & prostate.

I will also perform ABGs, Serum Calcium, Phosphate, ALP, PTH and Vitamin D_3 level.

I will assess his diabetic status by doing Fasting & Random Blood Sugar and HbA1c.

As he doesn't have any acute complication like acute pulmonary edema, he can be managed as outpatient.

For HT, I would like to adjust the doses of his medications, preferably a combination ARB and CCB.

I will prescribe α-1 hydroxycholecalciferol (if vitamin D deficient), along with calcium supplements, preferably as calcium carbonate.

I will refer the patient to the Nephrologist for further work-up and management including RRT.

I will identify and manage the risk factors like infection, obstruction, hypercalcemia, hyperuricemia, and will avoid the NSAIDSs & nephrotoxic drugs (and will adjust and monitor the doses of renally excreted medications).

I will suggest his GP to assess the response to treatment by regular monitoring of his BP, diabetic status, and renal functions.

I will address his social, occupational and dietary needs including the lifestyle changes.

I would like to arrange an early appointment with a Nephrologist and GP visit as required.

HISTORY

The following points are to be given special emphasis in the history:

Diabetic nephropathy: At what age the diabetes was diagnosed. How it presented (polyuria, polydipsia, weight loss, DKA or asymptomatic hyperglycemia /glycosuria). Ask about the renal involvement like dysuria, edema, HT, hypoglycemic events or control of diabetes and medications.

Hypertensive nephropathy: Duration, age of onset, how it was diagnosed, drugs, compliance, control & complications of disease and drugs like ACE-I /ARBs, family history. In women the history of pregnancy induced HT, pre-eclampsia /eclampsia.

Glomerulonephritis: Ask about generalized body swelling (Nephrotic /Nephritic, hematuria, proteinuria, oliguria, upper respiratory tract infections (sore throat & fever), sepsis, rash, hemoptysis, arthritis. Ask in details about the lab work-up and any renal biopsy report. Take the drug history like antihypertensive, immunosuppressive, NSAIDs use and dialysis therapy.

Polycystic Kidney Disease: How the disease was diagnosed (loin pain, hematuria, HT, polyuria, renal calculi, headache, intracranial bleed or visual disturbance (intracranial aneurysms), duration, family history.

Analgesic Nephropathy: Take the history of NSAIDs

type, dose, duration. Hematuria, HT, renal colic, GI bleeding, carcinoma, anemia.

Reflux nephropathy: Ask about recurrent urinary tract infection (UTI) since early childhood, urinary abnormality, enuresis, cystoscopy, urological interventions and frequent antibiotics use.

Connective tissue disorder: History of rash, arthritis, edema, HT (SLE, scleroderma), treatment and progression to ESRD (rapid or prolonged course).

Obstructive uropathy: Ask about congenital anomalies of genitourinary system in the young and due to prostate diseases, malignancy and stones in adults. Ask about ultrasound, other imaging studies and any previous urological interventions.

Treatment: What conservative management the patient is taking, dietary proteins, salt and fluid intake, lab reports like FBC, RFTs, USG, Renal biopsy. Medications (phosphate binders, active vitamin D3, Iron, antihypertensives, antidiabetics with diabetic control and hypoglycemic events, EPO with dose and duration, QoL related to anemia.

Ask about the mode of dialysis, duration, frequency, QoL on dialysis and any complications. Access for dialysis e.g. AVF, double lumen catheter or peritoneal catheter. Ask about transplantations, donor, living or cadaveric, related or unrelated. Post-transplant course,

QoL, medications & side-effects, and complications (infections, rejections, HT, new onset diabetes, neoplasms and medications, side-effects like hyperlipidemia, cosmetic effects, osteoporosis and fractures)

Socio-economic history: Ask about social history, employment, family arrangements, travels, sports, sexual function and economic situation.

If on conservative management: Ask about symptoms of anemia, renal osteodystrophy, gout, cardiac (cardiac failure, pericarditis, angina/MI), HT, cerebrovascular disease, gastritis, GERD, peripheral neuropathy, nutritional status, pruritus, restless legs syndrome and sleep.

If on dialysis: Ask about infections, hypotension, AVF (blockage, aneurysm, rupture), hypoglycemia, cardiac arrhythmias and seizures.

If had transplant: Ask about infections (viral like CMV, BKV), rejection (fever, graft pain or swelling), urinary leaks and obstruction. In patients with long-standing transplant ask about renal function, chronic rejection (proteinuria), recurrent GN, skin carcinomas, osteoporosis and fractures.

CLINICAL EXAMINATION

The following points are to be given special emphasis during examination:

GPE: General appearance, pallor, sallow color, emaciation, wasting, hydration, mental state, dyspnea, acidotic breathing, encephalopathy or coma.

Pulse and BP (Supine and standing).

Hands: Nails for anemia, half & half nails of hypoalbuminemia, tremors, pallor at palm crease, AVF, vasculitis, gangrene, neuropathy, wasting.

Arms: AVF, bruises, scratch marks, calcifications, and myopathy.

Face: Pallor, jaundice, rash, saddle-shaped nose, fetor.

Neck: JVP, double lumen catheter or its scar marks

Chest: Pericardial rub, pleural /pericardial effusion, cardiac failure, lung infection (consolidation), pacemaker, double lumen catheter or its scar marks.

Abdomen: Palpable kidneys (PKD, hydronephrosis, Fabry disease), graft scar, peritoneal catheter, bruit, hepato-splenomegaly, lymph nodes, ascites, bladder mass.

Digital rectal examination (DRE) for prostate, masses and blood loss.

Lower limbs: Edema, neuropathy, gout, myopathy, calcifications, rash, bruising, scratch marks, femoral catheters or AVF, pigmentation.

Back: Sacral edema, pressure sores.

DISCUSSION

Any aspect of CKD e.g. etiology, management, complications or renal replacement therapy (RRT) i.e. dialysis /transplantation can be asked with special emphasis on indications, modes, and complications of RRT in details.

Some hints are given below to tackle all these questions asked during discussion.

CHRONIC KIDNEY DISEASE

C hronic kidney disease (CKD) is defined as the evidence of kidney damage or decreased kidney function (GFR <60 ml/min/1.73m^2 or urinary albumin excretion ≥30 mg/day) for more than three months.

Classification or staging of CKD provides a guide for its management, prognosis and complications.

According to the Kidney Disease Improving Global Outcomes (KDIGO) 2012 guidelines; staging of CKD is done on the basis of the cause, GFR and albuminuria.

CRITERIA FOR CHRONIC KIDNEY DISEASE

	Either of the following for >3 months
Markers of kidney damage (one or more)	• Albuminuria (AER ≥30 mg/24 h) • ACR ≥30mg/g (≥3 mg/mmol)) • Urine sediment abnormalities • Electrolytes and other abnormalities due to tubular disorders • Abnormalities detected by histology • Structural abnormalities detected by imaging • History of kidney transplantation
Decreased GFR	<60 ml/min per 1.73 m^2

CKD CLASSIFICATION BASED ON GFR AND ALBUMINURIA

GFR stages	GFR (mL/min/1.73 m^2)	Terms
G1	≥90	Normal or high
G2	60 to 89	Mildly decreased
G3a	45 to 59	Mildly to moderately decreased
G3b	30 to 44	Moderately to severely decreased
G4	15 to 29	Severely decreased
G5	<15	Kidney failure (add D if treated by dialysis)
Albu-minuria stages	AER (mg/day)	
A1	<30	Normal to mildly increased
A2	30 to 300	Moderately increased
A3	>300	Severely increased (may be subdivided into nephrotic and non-nephrotic for DD, management, and risk prediction)

COMMON CAUSES OF RENAL FAILURE

- DM
- HT
- Vascular disease: RAS
- Glomerular disease: Primary /Secondary
- Chronic pyelonephritis
- Vasculitides
- Tubulo-Interstitial disease
- Congenital defects: PKD
- Myeloma
- Progression of AKI

FACTORS WHICH AGGRAVATE RENAL IMPAIRMENT

1. Infection
2. Obstruction
3. Dehydration
4. Intravascular volume depletion
5. Uncontrolled DM
6. Uncontrolled HT
7. Hypoxia
8. Hyperuricemia
9. Hypercalcemia
10. Anemia
11. Nephrotoxic Drugs: Aminoglycosides, NSAIDs, anti-cancer, anti-retroviral, Calcineurin-inhibitors, iodinated contrast agents.

INVESTIGATIONS

- FBC, U&Es
- Creatinine, eGFR
- Urinalysis, C/S
- ABGs
- LFTs, Serum albumin
- Serum protein electrophoresis
- Lipid profile
- Serum calcium, PO_4, ALP, PTH, Vitamin D3 level
- Hepatitis B, C and HIV screening

Imaging studies:

USG: For kidney size, cortex size and cortico-medullary differentiation to rule out AKI or obstructive uropathy.

CT scan: For renal cysts, masses, stones, retroperitoneal fibrosis.

MRI: Patients who cannot use contrast in CT especially in renal vein thrombosis.

Radionuclide scanning: Dimercapto succinic acid (DMSA) is static imaging and detects the structure while Diethylene triamine penta acetate (DTPA) and Mercaptoacetyltriglycine (MAG3) are dynamic imaging and assess the function.

COMPLICATIONS ASSOCIATED WITH CKD

ANEMIA

It is multifactorial but the two major factors are iron and EPO deficiency. It is usually normocytic normochromic.

New horizon has opened with the identification of hypoxia-inducible factor as one of the key regulators that control how cells respond to hypoxic conditions. It enhances the kidney and hepatic EPO synthesis and iron uptake from the intestine and opposes the deleterious effects of hepcidin (implicated in the pathophysiology of EPO resistant anemia). Prolyl-hydroxylase inhibitor prevents its degradation, allowing the stimulation of EPO gene expression in the kidneys.

MINERAL BONE DISORDER

CKD is usually associated with mineral bone disorder (MBD) and presents with hypocalcaemia, hyperphosphatemia, high PTH, osteopenia or osteoporosis and low vitamin-D called renal osteodystrophy due to secondary hyperparathyroidism.

Don't routinely prescribe vitamin D supplements, in the absence of suspected or documented deficiency, to suppress the elevated PTH levels in patients not on dialysis. Don't prescribe bisphosphonate with GFR <30 without a strong clinical rationale.

MANAGEMENT

- Identification and treatment of the cause
- Identification and treatment of aggravating factors
- Treatment of complications
- Preparation for dialysis and transplantation

Protein restriction: Avoid high protein diet and keep the daily intake to 0.8 g/kg body wt.

Salt restriction: Reduce the daily salt intake to <5 g sodium chloride (<2 g of Na).

Life-style changes:

- Physical activity compatible with CV health (at least 30 min five times a week).
- Optimize the weight (BMI 20–25 kg/m²)
- Stop smoking.

Hyperuricemia: There is insufficient evidence to support or refute the use of drugs to lower uric acid in CKD.

MANAGEMENT OF AGGRAVATING FACTORS

Renal hypoperfusion: All causes of renal hypoperfusion or hypovolemia (vomiting, diarrhea, diuretics, bleeding), hypotension and septicemia should be treated aggressively. .

Urinary tract obstruction: The cause of urinary tract obstruction such as renal stones, neoplasms, benign prostatic hyperplasia (BPH) and bladder outlet obstruction must be considered and treated.

Metabolic acidosis: When serum bicarbonate is <22 mmol/l, oral sodium bicarbonate supplements should be given to maintain it in the normal range (22-28 mmol/l).

High serum bicarbonate level within the normal range prevents the progression of CKD.

Infection: Patients with CKD are prone to infections due to low immunity. Influenza and pneumococcal vaccines are offered especially in elderly.

MANAGEMENT OF COMPLICATIONS

Volume overload:

Sodium and fluid restriction.

Loop diuretics.

Hyperkalemia:

Low potassium diet.

Avoid drugs causing hyperkalemia (ACE-I/ARBs).

In hperkalemic emergency (serum K^+ >6 mmol/l):

- IV Calcium gluconate to prevent arrhythmias.

- Salbutamol nebulization

- Insulin infusion with 50% glucose

- Loop diuretics if renal function not severely impaired

- Resin exchange, Dialysis

Mineral bone disorders:

For hyperphosphatemia, restrict dietary phosphate and administer phosphate binders to block its absorption from the intestine e.g. Calcium based phosphate binders or Sevelamer acetate or Carbonate.

Hypocalcemia can be treated with oral calcium supplements and active vitamin D3 analogues.

Osteoporosis prophylaxis.

Anemia: Correction of iron deficiency and EPO.

Hyperlipidemia: Statins

Pericarditis:

An indication for urgent dialysis.

Indomethacin and colchicine are effective to prevent the recurrence of pericarditis.

PREPARATION FOR RRT AND TRANSPLANT

The timing for initiation of dialysis is not universally agreed. However in patients with e-GFR 8-10 ml/min/1.73m² for non-diabetic and 15 ml/min/1.73m² for diabetics, dialysis should be started to avoid life-threatening complications.

Most CKD patients are in a denial phase for initiation of dialysis that needs multiple counseling sessions with the patient and the family.

Conservative management can be discussed with patients who don't opt for RRT.

Until transplant they must be on dialysis as a bridge to transplantation.

Preparation for HD requires an access like double lumen catheter, AVF or AV graft.
For PD Tenchkoff's catheter should be inserted below the umbilicus into the peritoneal cavity.

CKD AND MEDICATIONS

Temporarily discontinue the potentially nephrotoxic drugs and those with predominant renal excretion in patients with serious intercurrent illness which increases the risk of AKI, such as RAAS blockers (ACE-Is, ARBs, aldosterone inhibitors, renin inhibitors), diuretics, NSAIDs, metformin, lithium, and digoxin.

Metformin can be continued with GFR ≥45 ml/min; reviewed at 30–44 and discontinued at <30 ml/min/1.73m².

GFR should be considered when adjusting the doses of medications.

Patients taking potentially nephrotoxic agents such as lithium and Calcineurin inhibitors (cyclosporine, tacrolimus) should have GFR, electrolytes, and drug levels regularly monitored.

CKD patients should not be denied treatment for other conditions such as cancer but there should be appropriate dose adjustment of drugs according to the GFR.

RENAL REPLACEMENT THERAPY

R enal replacement therapy is offered to patients with ESRD and includes:

- Hemodialysis (HD)
- Peritoneal dialysis (PD)
- Renal transplantation

INDICATIONS FOR DIALYSIS

According to KDIGO guidelines, dialysis can be initiated when one or more of the following are present. This often occurs with GFR (5-10 ml/min).

- Symptoms or signs related to kidney failure (serositis, acid-base or electrolyte abnormalities, pruritus).
- Inability to control volume status or BP.
- Progressive deterioration in nutritional status refractory to dietary intervention.
- Cognitive impairment like encephalopathy

INDICATIONS FOR URGENT DIALYSIS

- Acute pulmonary edema
- Pericarditis
- Hyperkalemia resistant to medical therapy

TYPES OF DIALYSIS

- Hemodialysis
- Peritoneal dialysis

HEMODIALYSIS

Patients with GFR <30 ml/min should be immunized against hepatitis B and the response confirmed by checking anti-HBs antibody titer.

Complications:

- **Infection:** HIV, Hepatitis B/C, Bacterial
- **Electrolyte imbalance**
- **Hypotension**
- **Vascular access problems:** Bleeding, Thrombosis, Infection, Vascular insufficiency.
- **Dialysis arthropathy:** Amyloid formation especially in shoulders and wrists, due to accumulation of β2-microglobulin on long-standing HD.
- **Aluminum toxicity:** Dementia ± bone disease similar to osteomalacia can be prevented by using aluminum-free dialysate and avoiding aluminum-containing phosphate binders. It is rare now-a-days

PERITONEAL DIALYSIS

It is based on the principal of diffusion and osmosis where peritoneal membrane acts as a dialyzer and exchange occurs between the blood and dialysis solution in the peritoneal cavity.

It has advantages over HD as it can be done at home by the patient himself, no machine is involved, no anticoagulation, no danger of transmission of HBV/HCV/HIV, more liberal protein intake, no hypotension, better preservation of residual renal function, less amount of EPO needed and can avoid exposure to infections.

Commonly used techniques of PD:
- **Intermittent peritoneal dialysis (IPD):**

Mainly used in AKI in hemodynamically unstable patients especially in children & elderly and where facility for HD is not available.
- **Continuous ambulatory peritoneal dialysis (CAPD):**

Tenchkoff's catheter is placed permanently in the peritoneal cavity subcutaneously or by laparoscopic or open surgery. Dialysate bags are used with exchanges up to 4 times a day. Automated PD with a cycler machine can also be used with the same principle.

Contraindications:
- Abdominal sepsis
- Anti-coagulant therapy
- Respiratory failure
- Previous abdominal surgery

Complications:
- Peritonitis
- Catheter blockage
- Weight gain
- Poor diabetic control
- Lactic acidosis
- Pleural effusion
- Leakage

RENAL TRANSPLANTATION

End Sate Kidney Disease (ESRD) is the only indication for renal transplantation. This gold standard treatment of ESRD should be considered at GFR <20 ml/min/1.73m² and evidence of progressive and irreversible CKD over the preceding 6–12 months.
It can be living or cadaveric.

CONTRAINDICATIONS

Absolute:

- Active infection
- Active malignancy
- Active substance abuse
- Reversible renal failure
- Psychiatric illness
- Poor compliance

Relative:

Systemic conditions like malnutrition, primary oxalosis, peripheral vascular disease, morbid obesity and systemic amyloidosis.

PRE-TRANSPLANT WORK-UP

Blood group, HLA tissue-typing and cross-match between donor and recipient.

POST-TRANSPLANT IMMUNOSUPPRESSION

Calcineurin inhibitors (cyclosporine, tacrolimus), anti-proliferative (AZA, MMF) and steroids.

POST-TRANSPLANT COMPLICATIONS

- Acute graft rejection
- Urological complications: Urinoma, lymphocele, ureteric obstruction at ureteric anastomosis
- Persistent HT
- Cyclosporine-induced nephrotoxicity
- Complications of immunosuppression:

    - Opportunistic infections: viral (CMV, BK virus), bacterial, fungal

    - Skin malignancy
- NODAT
- PTLD
- Atherosclerosis
- Recurrence of primary glomerulonephritis

LAND-MARK TRIALS

· RENAAL
Reduction of Endpoints in NIDDM with Angiotensin II Antagonist Losartan

> Inhibiting RAAS in patients with T2M and CKD reduces the proteinuria and preserves the renal function.

In this RCT, 1513 patients with DM and nephropathy were randomized to losartan 50-100 mg/day or placebo in addition to conventional antihypertensive treatment and followed for 3.4 years.

The primary outcome was the composite of a doubling of base-line serum creatinine, ESRD disease, or death. Secondary end-points included a composite of morbidity and mortality from CV causes, proteinuria, and the rate of progression of renal disease.

A total of 327 patients in losartan group reached the primary end-point, as compared to 359 in placebo group (risk reduction, 16%; P=0.02).

Losartan reduced the incidence of doubling of serum creatinine (risk reduction, 25%; P=0.006) and ESRD (risk reduction, 28%; P=0.002) but had no effect on the rate of death. The benefit exceeded that attributable to changes in BP.

The composite of morbidity and mortality from CV causes was similar in two groups, although the rate of first hospitalization for heart failure was significantly lower with losartan (risk reduction, 32%; P=0.005). The level of proteinuria declined by 35% with losartan (P<0.001).

Ref: N Engl J Med 2001; 345:861-9.

• MDRD
Modification of Diet in Renal Disease

In moderate renal insufficiency, low-protein diet has a small benefit. While in severe renal insufficiency, a very-low-protein, as compared to low-protein diet, doesn't significantly slow the progression of disease. Patients in low-BP group with more pronounced proteinuria at base-line has significantly slower rate of decline in GFR.

In this RCT, 840 patients with various chronic renal diseases were investigated for dietary interventions and followed for 2.2 years.

In study-1, 585 patients with GFR 25-55 ml/min were randomly assigned to usual-protein or low-protein diet (1.3 or 0.58 g/kg body wt/day) and to a usual or low-BP group (mean BP, 107 or 92 mmHg).

In study-2, 255 patients with GFR 13-24 ml/min were randomly assigned to low-protein (0.58 g/kg/day) or very-low protein diet (0.28 g/kg/day) with a keto amino acid supplement, and a usual or low-BP group.

In study-1, the projected mean decline in GFR at 3 years did not differ significantly between the diet or BP groups. As compared with usual-protein and usual-BP group, the low-protein and low-BP group had more rapid decline in GFR during the first 4 months and a slower decline thereafter.

In study-2, the very-low-protein group had marginally slower decline in GFR than low-protein group (P=0.07). There was no delay in time to occurrence of ESRD or death.

In both studies, patients in low-BP group with more pronounced proteinuria at base-line had significantly slower rate of decline in GFR.

Ref: New Eng J Med. 1994; 330:877-84.

TRIALS ON PERITONEAL DIALYSIS

• CANUSA study

Canada-USA Peritoneal Dialysis Study

> Increasing the dose of peritoneal dialysis is associated with improved survival of patients.

This was a prospective cohort study of 680 consecutive patients commencing peritoneal dialysis in 14 centers in Canada and USA with follow-up period of 3 years.

There were 90 deaths, 137 transplants, and 118 technique failures. Fifteen withdrew from dialysis. The relative risk (RR) of death increased with increased age, insulin-dependent DM, CV disease, decreased serum albumin and worsened nutritional status.

A decrease of 0.1 unit Kt/V per week was associated with 5% increase in RR of death; a decrease of 5 L/1.73m² CrCl/week was associated with 7% increase in RR of death. The RR of technique failure was increased with decreased albumin and CCr. Hospitalization was increased with decreased serum albumin, worsened nutrition according to subjective global assessment and decreased CCr. A weekly Kt/V of 2.1 and CCr of 70 L/1.73 m² were each associated with an expected 2-yr survival of 78%.

Ref: J Am Soc Nephrol 1996; 7:198-207.

. ADEMEX
Adequacy of PD in Mexico

Increase in peritoneal small-solute clearance has neutral effect on patient survival, even when the groups are stratified according to the factors known to affect survival.

In this RCT, 965 patients were randomly assigned to intervention or control group. Control group continued preexisting PD prescription (Four daily exchanges with 2L of standard PD solution). Intervention group was treated with modified prescription, to achieve peritoneal creatinine clearance (pCCr) of 60 L/wk/1.73 m^2 and followed for 2 years.

In control group, pCrCl and urea clearance (Kt/V) remained constant for the duration of study. In intervention group, pCrCl and Kt/V predictably increased and remained separated from the values for control group for entire duration of study (p<0.01).

Patient survival was similar for control and intervention groups in intent-to-treat analysis, with RR of death (intervention/control) of 1.00 [95% CI, 0.80 to 1.24]. Overall, control group exhibited 1-yr survival of 85.5% (CI, 82.2 to 88.7%) and 2-yr survival 68.3% (CI, 64.2 to 72.9%). Intervention group 1-yr survival 83.9% (CI, 80.6 to 87.2%) and 2-yr 69.3% (CI, 65.1 to 73.6%). An as-treated analysis revealed similar results (overall RR=0.93; CI, 0.71 to 1.22; p=0.61).

Mortality rates remained similar even after adjustment for factors known to be associated with survival for patients undergoing PD (age, DM, S. albumin, normalized protein equivalent of total nitrogen appearance, and anuria).

Ref: J Am Soc Nephrol 2002; 13:1307-20.

• HONG KONG study

In CAPD patients total Kt/V don't significantly affect survival. However, it should be maintained above 1.7.

In this RCT, 320 new CAPD patients with baseline renal Kt/V <1.0 were randomized into three Kt/V targets: group A, 1.5 to 1.7; group B, 1.7 to 2.0; and group C, >2.0. The nutritional status was assessed every 6 months and dialysis prescription adjusted accordingly. The follow-up period was 24.3 months. Nutritional assessment included serum albumin and composite nutritional index (CNI). Patients were allowed to withdraw at the discretion of their physicians or themselves.

There was no statistical difference in survival among three groups. However, there were more patients withdrawn by physicians in group A (group A, 16; group B, 7; and group C, 6; P= 0.02). There was no difference in serum albumin, CNI scores, and hospitalization rate, but there were more patients in group A requiring EPO treatment.

Ref: Kidney Int 2003; 64:649-56.

TRIALS ON HEMODIALYSIS

. NCDS
National Cooperative Dialysis Study

> Morbidity in patients on HD may be decreased by prescriptions with more efficient removal of urea if dietary intake of protein and other nutrients is adequate.

This was the first major RCT on HD dose comparing high vs. low BUN targets and short and long duration of HD.

In this study, 151 patients were evaluated for the clinical effects of different dialysis prescriptions. Four treatment groups were divided along two dimensions: dialysis treatment time (long or short), and BUN averaged with respect to time (TAC_{urea}) (high or low). The dietary protein was not restricted.

There was no difference in mortality between the groups. Withdrawal of patients from high-BUN groups for medical reasons was significantly greater than low BUN groups. Hospitalization was also greater in high-BUN groups, but dialysis treatment time had no significant effects.

Ref: N Engl J Med 1981; 305:1176–81.

◆ HEMO study
Hemodialysis study

> Patients undergoing hemodialysis thrice weekly appear to have no major benefit from a higher dialysis dose.
> There was no difference in survival with high dose or high flux dialysis.

In this RCT, 1846 patients undergoing thrice-weekly hemodialysis, were assigned randomly to standard or high dose of dialysis and to a low-flux or high-flux dialyzer.

In standard-dose group, the mean urea-reduction ratio was $66.3\pm2.5\%$, the single-pool Kt/V was 1.32 ± 0.09, and the equilibrated Kt/V was 1.16 ± 0.08; in high-dose group, the values were $75.2\pm2.5\%$, 1.71 ± 0.11, and 1.53 ± 0.09, respectively.

Flux, estimated on the basis of $beta_2$-microglobulin clearance, was 3 ± 7 ml/min in low-flux group and 34 ± 11 ml/min in high-flux group.

The primary outcome, death from any cause, was not significantly influenced by the dose or flux assignment: RR of death in high-dose group as compared with standard-dose group was 0.96 (95% CI, 0.84 to 1.10; P=0.53), and RR of death in high-flux group as compared with low-flux group was 0.92 (95% CI, 0.81 to 1.05; P=0.23).

The main secondary outcomes (first hospitalization for cardiac causes or death from any cause, first hospitalization for infection or death from any cause, first 15% decrease in serum albumin or death from any cause, and all hospitalizations not related to vascular access) also did not differ significantly between either the dose or the flux groups. Possible benefits of dose or flux interventions were suggested in two of seven prespecified subgroups of patients.

Ref: N Engl J Med 2002; 347:2010-9.

TRIALS ON RENAL TRANSPLANT

. FREEDOM

In renal transplant patients receiving cyclosporine, mycophenolate and basiliximab induction, no steroids or withdrawal at day 7 achieves comparable 1-year renal function to a standard steroid regimen.

In this randomized, open-label, multicenter study, 336 de novo renal transplant patients were assigned to no steroids, steroids to day 7, or standard steroids, with cyclosporine, mycophenolate and basiliximab and followed for 12 months.

The median 12-month GFR was not significantly different in steroid-free or steroid-withdrawal groups (58.6 ml/min/1.73m^2 and 59.1 mL/min/1.73m^2 versus standard steroids (60.8 mL/min/1.73m^2. The incidence of biopsy-proven acute rejection (BPAR), graft loss or death was 36% in steroid-free group (p=0.007 vs. standard steroids), 29.6% with steroid withdrawal (N.S) and 19.3% with standard steroids. BPAR was significantly less frequent with standard steroids than either of the other two regimens. Reduced de novo use of antidiabetic and lipid-lowering medication, triglycerides and weight gain were observed in one or both steroid-minimization group versus standard steroids.

Ref: Am J Transplant 2008; 8:307-16.

Erratum in Am J Transplant 2008; 8:1080.

• BENEFIT
Belatacept Evaluation of Nephroprotection and Efficacy as First-line Immunosuppression Trial

> Belatacept is associated with superior renal function and similar patient and graft survival post-transplant as compared to cyclosporine, despite a higher rate of early acute rejection.

Belatacept, a costimulation blocker, may preserve renal function and improve long-term outcomes versus calcineurin inhibitors (CNI) in kidney transplantation. This Phase III study assessed a more intensive (MI) or less intensive (LI) regimen of belatacept versus cyclosporine in adults receiving a kidney transplant from living or standard criteria deceased donors. The co-primary endpoints at 12 months were patient/graft survival, a composite renal impairment endpoint (percent with a measured GFR <60 mL/min/1.73 m^2 at Month 12 or a decrease in mGFR $\geq$10 mL/min/1.73 m^2 Month 3 - Month 12) and the incidence of acute rejection.

At Month 12, both belatacept regimens had similar patient/graft survival versus cyclosporine (MI: 95%, LI: 97% and cyclosporine: 93%), and were associated with superior renal function as measured by composite renal impairment endpoint (MI: 55%; LI: 54% and cyclosporine: 78%; p $\leq$0.001 MI or LI versus cyclosporine) and by mGFR (65, 63 and 50 mL/min for MI, LI and cyclosporine; p$\leq$0.001 MI or LI versus cyclosporine). Belatacept patients experienced a higher incidence (MI: 22%, LI: 17% and cyclosporine: 7%) and grade of acute rejection episodes.

Safety was generally similar, but PTLD was more common in belatacept groups.

Ref: Am J Transplant 2010;10:535-46.

• BENEFIT - EXT

Belatacept-treated patients maintained a high rate of patient and graft survival comparable to cyclosporine-treated patients, despite an early increased occurrence of acute rejection and PTLD.

The clinical profile of belatacept in kidney transplant recipients was evaluated to determine if earlier results in BENEFIT study were sustained at 3 years.

A total of 92% (MI), 92% (LI), and 89% (cyclosporine) patients survived with a functioning graft. The mean calculated GFR (cGFR) was ~ 21 mL/min/1.73 m^2 higher in belatacept groups versus cyclosporine at year 3.

From month 3 to 36, the mean cGFR increased in belatacept groups by +1.0 ml/min per year (MI) and +1.2 mL/min/year (LI) versus a decline of -2.0 ml/min/

year (cyclosporine). One cyclosporine-treated patient experienced acute rejection between year 2 and 3. There were no new safety signals and no new PTLD cases after month 18.

Ref: Am J Transplant 2012; 12:210-7.

• HARMONY
Rabbit-ATG or Basiliximab induction for rapid steroid withdrawal after renal transplantation

> Rapid steroid withdrawal after induction-therapy in renal transplantation can be achieved without loss of efficacy and is advantageous in regards to incidence of post-transplantation diabetes.

Standard practice for immunosuppressive therapy after renal transplantation is quadruple therapy using antibody induction, low-dose tacrolimus, MMF mofetil, and corticosteroids. Long-term steroids significantly increase the CV risk with negative effects on outcome, especially post-transplantation diabetes, associated with morbidity and mortality.

In this open-label, multicentre, RCT, 615 renal transplant recipients were randomly assigned to either basiliximab induction with low-dose tacrolimus, MMF, and steroid maintenance therapy (arm A), rapid corticosteroid withdrawal on day 8 (arm B), or rapid corticosteroid withdrawal on day 8 after rabbit ATG (arm C).

Follow-up period was 12 months.

BPAR rates were not reduced by rabbit ATG (9·9%) compared with either treatment arm A (11·2%) or B (10·6%). Rapid steroid withdrawal reduced post-transplantation diabetes in arm B to 24% and arm C 23% compared with 39% in control arm A (A versus B and C: p=0·0004). Patient survival (94·7% in arm A, 97·4% arm B, and 96·9% in arm C) and censored graft survival (96·1% in arm A, 96·8% arm B, and 95·8% in arm C) after 12 months were excellent and equivalent in all arms. Safety parameters such as infections or post-transplantation malignancies did not differ between the study arms.

Ref: Lancet. 2016; 388:3006-16.

• TRANSFORM
TRANSplant eFficacy and safety Outcomes with an eveRolimus-based regiMen

EVR+rCNI regimen offers comparable efficacy and graft function with low tBPAR and dnDSA rates and significantly lower incidence of viral infections relative to standard-of-care.

In this prospective, open-label trial, 2037 de novo renal transplant recipients were randomized to everolimus (EVR) with reduced-exposure calcineurin inhibitor (EVR+rCNI) or MMF with standard-exposure CNI and followed for 2 years.

Non-inferiority of EVR+rCNI regimen for primary endpoint of treated biopsy-proven acute rejection (tBPAR) or eGFR<50 mL/min/1.73m^2 was achieved (47.9% vs 43.7%; difference=4.2%; 95% CI= -0.3, 8.7; P=.006). Mean eGFR was stable up to month 24 (52.6 vs 54.9 ml/min/1.73m^2) in both arms. The incidence of de novo donor-specific antibodies (dnDSA) was lower in EVR +rCNI arm (12.3% vs 17.6%). Although discontinuation rates due to adverse events were higher with EVR+rCNI (27.2% vs 15.0%), rates of CMV (2.8% vs 13.5%) and BK virus (5.8% vs 10.3%) infections were lower. CMV infection rates were significantly lower with EVR+rCNI even in the D+/R- high-risk group (P<0.0001).

Ref: Am J Transplant 2019; 19:3018-34.

TRIALS ON ANEMIA IN CRF

• CREATE

In patients with CKD, early complete correction of anemia does not reduce the risk of CV events.

In this study, 603 patients with eGFR 15 to 35 ml/min/1.73 m² and mild-to-moderate anemia (Hb 11 to 12.5 g/dl) were studied to a target Hb value in the normal range (13 to 15 g/dl, group 1) or the subnormal range (10.5 to 11.5 g/dL, group 2). EPO was initiated at randomization (group 1) or only after Hb level fell <10.5 g/dL (group 2). Follow-up period was 3 years.

Complete correction of anemia did not affect the likelihood of first CV event (58 events in group 1 vs. 47 in group 2; hazard ratio, 0.78; 95% CI, 0.53 to 1.14; P=0.2). LV mass index remained stable in both groups. The mean eGFR was 24.9 ml/min in group 1 and 24.2 ml/min in group 2 at baseline and decreased by 3.6 and 3.1 ml/min per year, respectively (P=0.4). Dialysis was required in more patients in group 1 than group 2 (127 vs. 111, P=0.03). General health and physical function improved significantly (P=0.003 and P<0.001, respectively, in group 1 as compared to group 2).

There was no significant difference in combined incidence of adverse events between the two groups, but hypertensive episodes and headaches were more prevalent in group 1.

Ref: New Engl J Med 2006; 355:2071-84.

• CHOIR
Correction of Anemia with Epoetin Alfa in Chronic Kidney disease

> In CKD patients with anemia, treating with EPO to a lower Hb target as compared to higher is associated with reduced CV events, stroke, hospitalization and death.

In this open-label trial, 1432 patients with CKD were randomly assigned to receive a dose of EPO targeted to achieve Hb level of 13.5 g/dl or 11.3 g/dl. The median study duration was 16 months.

A total of 222 composite events occurred; 125 in high Hb group, and 97 in low Hb group (hazard ratio, 1.34; 95% CI, 1.03 to 1.74; P=0.03). There were 65 deaths (29.3%), 101 hospitalizations for CCF (45.5%), 25 MI (11.3%), and 23 strokes (10.4%). Seven patients (3.2%) were hospitalized for CCF and MI combined, and one patient (0.5%) died after having a stroke. Improvements in QoL were similar in the two groups. More patients in high Hb group had at least one serious adverse event.

Ref: N Engl J Med 2006; 355:2085-98.

· DRIVE
Dialysis Patients' Response to IV Iron with Elevated ferritin

Administration of IV Iron is superior to no iron therapy in anemic dialysis patients receiving adequate EPO and having ferritin >500 ng/ml and TSAT <25%.

In this RCT, 134 patients with CKD on maintenance HD, Hb <11 g/dl, ferritin >500 ng/ml, TSAT <25%, and on adequate EPO dosage, were randomized to receive IV ferric gluconate versus no iron.

At 6 weeks, Hb increased significantly more (P= 0.028) in IV iron group (1.6 _ 1.3 g/dl) than control group (1.1 _ 1.4 g/dl). Hb response occurred faster (P=0.035) and more patients responded after IV iron than in control group (P= 0.041). Ferritin <800 or >800 ng/ml had no relationship to the magnitude or likelihood of responsiveness to IV iron relative to control group. Similarly, the superiority of IV iron compared with no iron was similar whether baseline TSAT was above or below the study median of 19%. Ferritin decreased in control subjects (174_225 ng/ml) and increased after IV iron (173 _272 ng/ml; P <0.001). IV iron resulted in a greater increase in TSAT than control subjects (7.5_7.4 *versus* 1.8_5.2%; P<0.001). Reticulocyte Hb content fell only in control subjects, suggesting worsening iron deficiency.

Ref: J Am Soc Nephrol 2007; 18:975–84.

• PIVOTAL

> In patients on HD, a proactive regimen of high dose IV
> iron is better than reactive regimen of low dose IV iron
> and results in lower doses of EPO administered.

In this multicenter, open-label trial with blinded end-point evaluation, 2141 patients with ESRD on maintenance HD were randomized to either a reactive strategy of low dose (0 to 400 mg monthly, with ferritin <200 µg/l or TSAT <20% being a trigger for iron administration) or proactive strategy of high dose IV iron sucrose (400 mg monthly, unless ferritin was >700 µg/l or TSAT ≥40%). The median follow-up was 2.1 years.

Patients in high-dose group received a median monthly iron dose of 264 mg (interquartile range [25th to 75th percentile], 200 to 336), as compared to 145 mg (inter-quartile range, 100 to 190) in low-dose group. The median monthly dose of ESA was 29,757 IU in high-dose and 38,805 IU in low-dose group (median difference, −7539 IU; 95% CI, −9485 to −5582).

A total of 320 patients (29.3%) in high-dose group had a primary end-point event, as compared with 338 (32.3%) in low-dose group (hazard ratio, 0.85; 95% CI, 0.73 to 1.00; P<0.001 for non-inferiority; P=0.04 for superiority).

In an analysis that used a recurrent-events approach, there were 429 events in high-dose and 507 in low-dose group (rate ratio, 0.77; 95% CI, 0.66 to 0.92). The infection rate was same in the two groups.

Ref: N Engl J Med 2019; 380:447-58.

• ROXADUSTAT study

> Hypoxia-inducible factor, propyl hydroxylase inhibitor, roxadustat is non-inferior to parenteral EPO in the treatment of anemia of CKD.

In this trial, 305 patients with CKD on dialysis were randomly assigned to oral roxadustat or parenteral EPO and followed for 26 weeks.

Roxadustat increased the transferrin level, maintained serum iron and attenuated decreases in transferrin saturation. The decrease in TC and LDL-C was greater with roxadustat than EPO. Roxadustat was associated with reduction in hepcidin as compared to EPO. Hyperkalemia and URTI occurred at a higher frequency in Roxadustat group, and HT occurred at a higher frequency in EPO group. Roxadustat led to a numerically greater mean change in Hb level from the baseline than EPO and was statistically non inferior.

Ref: N Engl J Med 2019; 381:1011-22.

CORONARY HEART DISEASE

P atients having coronary heart disease (CHD) can also be brought forward as long-cases in the clinical exams of Internal Medicine because of their easy availability and because they may also have DM &/or HT. These additional features make them a good case for discussion.

Dyslipidemia and even smoking can also be discussed along with CHD.

The summary and management plan of a typical case with CHD is given below:

SUMMARY

This gentleman, Mr. Khan, 60 years old, from Swat, shopkeeper by profession, is a known case of type 2 diabetes from the last 7 years - on oral hypoglycemic drugs. He is also having HT for 5 years and CHD for one year.

He is an ex-smoker with 20 pack years; quitted smoking a year back when he had ACS for which he got admission to the CCU in a tertiary care hospital.

This time he presented to A&E with shortness of breath - NYHA class III/IV and a sense of chest compression for 4 hours. After initial management at the casualty (with Loading doses of anti-platelets, O_2, IV Furosemide, and Parenteral Nitrates) he got better and was admitted to the Medical unit.

On examination my patient is sitting comfortably in the bed with some respiratory distress and has a cannula in the left arm. His pulse rate is 108 beats/min, regular, BP 145/100 mmHg, elevated JVP, bilateral pedal edema, S3 gallop rhythm and bilateral basal crackles.

He has got: **Type 2 diabetes, HT, Coronary heart disease with CCF.**

MANAGEMENT PLAN

I will perform an ECG, Chest x-ray, Echocardiography, and certain investigations like Trop T, Lipid profile, FBC, Blood sugar, and U&Es for the initial assessment.

I will carry on with the treatment of DM (preferably insulin), HT, CHD, and Heart failure.

I will refer the patient to the Cardiologist once he is stable for further assessment and necessary management.

I will identify and manage the risk factors like smoking, and hypercholesterolemia. I will manage for adequate control of diabetes, HT and prescribe the lipid lowering drugs.

I will arrange for the patient's counseling and education, and will suggest his GP to assess the response to treatment.

I will address his social, occupational, and dietary needs including lifestyle changes, exercise, and rehabilitation.

DISCUSSION

The discussion will mainly revolve around the risk factors for coronary heart disease, the management of acute coronary syndrome (ACS) and heart failure.

Some useful hints for the proper answers to the possible questions are given below.

Some of the trials in cardiology are quite popular and had provided the basis for the best clinical practices of the time. A brief summary of these landmark trials is given in the end. Reference to these trials should be given where appropriate during the discussion.

CORONARY HEART DISEASE

Myocardial ischemia due to reduced blood supply or demand-supply mismatch that commonly presents as chest pain. It is the leading cause of death worldwide. CHD can present as:

- Stable Angina
- ACS: STEMI
        Non-STEMI
        Unstable angina

In most of the cases myocardial ischemia is due to atherosclerotic disease of the coronary arteries but rarely, it may be due to:

- Structural heart disease (AS, HCM)
- Arrhythmia
- Severe anemia
- Shock
- Arteritis

RISK FACTORS

These can be "Modifiable" or "Non-modifiable".

Smoking, HT, and dyslipidemia are at the top of the list amongst the modifiable risk factors.

Non-modifiable:
- Age
- Ethnic background
- Family history of CHD

Modifiable:
- Smoking
- HT
- Dyslipidemia
- DM
- Physical inactivity
- Being overweight

CLINICAL CLASSIFICATION

OF CHEST PAIN

Typical angina (definite)	Meets three of the following characteristics: 1. Substernal chest discomfort of characteristic quality and duration 2. Provoked by exertion or emotional stress 3. Relieved by rest &/or nitroglycerine
Atypical angina (probable)	Meets two of the these characteristics
Non-cardiac chest pain	Meets one or none of the characteristics

ANGINA PECTORIS

Chest pain due to transient myocardial ichemia.

The pain is typically retrosternal, crushing, squeezing, choking or heaviness in character, radiating to the left arm, shoulder, neck, jaw, epigastrium and occasionally to the back.

It is brought on or exaggerated by exertion or anxiety and relieved by rest or sublingual GTN.

Angina pectoris is diffuse and cannot be localized to a single point. If there is no substantial change in the symptoms over several weeks it is labeled as stable angina.

INVESTIGATIONS

- Resting ECG
- ETT - Bruce protocol
- Echocardiography to rule out AS, HCM and look for LV

  systolic impairment
- Pharmacologic stress test (Dobutamine stress-echocardiography)
- Exercise echocardiography
- Exercise Radionuclide scan /Myocardial perfusion imaging
- CT /MR angiography
- Invasive coronary angiography

HIGH RISK FEATURES
- Accelerating symptoms in the last 48 hours
- Prolonged ongoing chest pain > 20 mins
- Pulmonary edema
- Hypotension, Brady or Tachycardia
- Sustained Ventricular arrhythmias
- Resting angina with dynamic ST/T changes
- Positive cardiac biomarkers (Trop I or T)

CANADIAN CARDIOVASCULAR SOCIETY (CCS) CLASSIFICATION OF ANGINA

CLASS	DESCRIPTION
I	Angina only during strenuous or prolonged physical activity
II	Slight limitation, with angina only during vigorous physical activity
III	Symptoms with everyday living activities, i.e. moderate limitation
IV	Inability to perform any activity without angina or angina at rest, i.e. severe limitation

MANAGEMENT

Non-pharmacologic:

- Lifestyle modifications
  Regular exercise 30 to 60 mins five times a week
  Optimize weight
  Low fat diet
- Avoid risk factors
  Smoking cessation, Control of DM, HT and dyslipidemia.
- Address psychological stress factors

Pharmacologic:

- Anti-platelet therapy (preferably Aspirin)
- β-blockers (Bisoprolol, Carvedilol, Metoprolol)
- Calcium channel blockers (Diltiazem)
- Nitrates (Isosorbide mononitrate or dinitrate)
- Lipid lowering agents (Statins)
- Coronary revascularization procedures (PCI / CABG)

UNSTABLE ANGINA

ngina is labeled as unstable if it is:
- New onset (<2 months duration)   or
- Increasing severity in frequency and duration (crescendo angina)   or
- Angina at rest (CCS class III/IV)

INVESTIGATIONS

- ECG
- Routine blood tests (FBC, U&Es, Lipid profile)
- Cardiac biomarkers (Troponin I and T)
- Bedside echocardiography
- Chest x-ray (to rule out other causes of chest pain)

MANAGEMENT

Unstable angina is a cardiac emergency and is included in the ACS.

The patient is admitted and started on parenteral nitrates along with anti-platelets, β-blocker, CCB (only when β-blockers are contraindicated and in suspected spastic angina), opioid analgesics for pain relief, parenteral anticoagulation (IV unfractionated heparin or IV and SC LMWH like enoxaparin) and an early coronary angiography with possible intervention.

ACUTE MYOCARDIAL INFARCTION

I schemic death of a portion of myocardium due to complete blockage of its blood supply. The most common cause of death in developed countries.

It is defined as a rise in the cardiac troponins with at least one value above the 99th percentile of the upper reference limit together with evidence of ischemia (symptoms, ECG, echocardiographic or other imaging evidence of myocardial ischemia).

ECG CHANGES IN ACUTE MI

There is ST deviation, appearance of Q-waves, and T wave inversion in acute MI.

In STEMI, the ECG changes are confined to the leads that face the infarct.

Inferior:	Leads II, III, aVF
Anterior:	Leads V2 to V5
High lateral:	Leads I and aVL
Anteroseptal:	Leads V1 to V3

Extensive anterolateral: V1 to V6 and Leads I, aVL

Right ventricular infarction: Isolated RV infarction is rare. It is usually associated with inferior MI, and affects the right ventricle. ECG shows ST elevations in V1 &/or aVR. The patient may present with shock and IV fluid challenge may be tried to elevate the BP. Right sided leads are recorded to confirm the diagnosis of RV infarction (V3R, V4R).

LATERAL (POSTERIOR) INFARCTION

Lateral infarction (formerly termed posterior or postero-lateral) infarction.

ECG shows dominant R waves and ST depression in leads V1 to V3.

Additional leads (posterior leads V7, V8, V9) on the posterior thorax are required to record the elevation of ST segment caused by transmural myocardial ischemia and the negative deviation of QRS complex caused by MI in this region.

CARDIAC BIO-MARKERS

Help to diagnose, evaluate and monitor the patients suspected of ACS.

ACUTE CARDIAC BIOMARKERS

BIO-MARKER	TIME TO INCREASE	REMAINS ELEVATED
Cardiac Troponins (Trop T & I)	3-4 hrs and peaks at 24-48 hrs	10-14 days
High sensitivity Cardiac Troponin	Within 3 hours	Same as above
CK-MB	4-6 hrs and peaks at 24 hrs	48-72 hours

Key: CK-MB – Myocardium specific creatinine kinase.

MANAGEMENT

IMMEDIATE

- Brief history and examination
- Get an ECG within 10 mins
- Bed rest
- Establish IV live
- Dispersible aspirin
- Oral platelet P2Y12 receptor antagonists (Clopidorel, Prasugrel, Ticagrelor)
- Nitrates to control elevated BP
- Beta blockers
- Parenteral anticoagulation
- O_2 inhalation if SaO2 <90%
- Relieve the pain with IV Opiods
- Reperfusion therapy (Thrombolysis/PCI)

CONTRAINDICATIONS TO THROMBOLYSIS

Absolute:

- Previous hemorrhagic stroke or ischemic stroke within 3 months
- Known intracranial neoplasm, structural cerebral vascular lesion or closed head injury within 3 months
- Active bleeding or bleeding diathesis
- Intracranial or intraspinal surgery within 2 months
- Severe uncontrolled HT BP > 180/110 unresponsive to medical therapy
- For SK - prior exposure within 6 months

Relative:

- Prolonged or traumatic CPR >10 mins
- History of ischemic stroke > 3 months
- Severe HT BP >180/110 mmHg at presentation
- Recent <3 weeks surgery or trauma
- Current use of oral anticoagulants
- Recent internal bleeding (2-4) weeks
- Pregnancy
- Active peptic ulcer

SUBSEQUENT IN-HOSPITAL MANAGEMENT

- Monitored in CCU for 48 to 72 hours.

- Aspirin 75-150 mg daily.

- $P2Y_{12}$ antagonist-Clopidogrel 75 mg daily

- β-blockers: (For all except those with decompensated heart failure, hypersensitivity to β-blockers, bronchial asthma and COPD)

- Lipid lowering medications (Statins)

- ACE-Is /ARBs

- Diuretics if symptoms of HF

- Nitrates for anginal symptoms and HF

- Oral Anticoagulants only if LV thrombus

- Adequate control of DM and HT

- Gradual mobilization

- Plan self-education, follow-up and rehabilitations after discharge

TREATMENT ON DISCHARGE

- Cardiac rehabilitation: Exercise, dietary advice.

- Address risk factors and modify if necessary.

- Keep BP <130/80 mm Hg.

- Lipid lowering therapy: (Statins as 1st line) aggressive LDL-C reduction to <70mg/dL or >50% reduction from baseline.

- Low dose Aspirin: to be given indefinitely.

- Oral platelet P2Y12 receptor antagonists (Clopidogrel 75 mg daily) for at least 12 months.

- ACE inhibitors: continued indefinitely for patients with LV dysfunction and CCF.

- Aldosterone antagonists: (spironolactone, Eplerenone) for patients with LV dysfunction.

- β-blockers: to be continued indefinitely.

- Diuretics: for patients with HF.

- Oral long-acting Nitrates.

- Review at 4-6 weeks.

RISK-STRATIFICATION

Certain scoring systems are used to calculate the in-hospital and 6 months mortality:

- TIMI Risk score
- GRACE Risk score

Procedures for risk stratification:

- Submaximal exercise tolerance test (70% of the target heart rate)
- Echocardiography
- Evoked potentials
- Holter monitor
- Angiography: For those with Non-STEMI and in whom sub-maximal stress test shows ischemia.
- Myocardial perfusion imaging (MPI) to look for stress induced ischemia and myocardium at risk.

COMPLICATIONS
OF ACUTE MI

Early:

- Arrythmias: Tachyarrythmias or heart blocks
- Heart failure or cardiogenic shock
- Early pericarditis
- Angina or recurrent infarction
- Thrombo-embolism (Stroke)
- MR, ventricular septal or free-wall rupture

Late:

- Post-MI syndrome (Dressler's syndrome)
- Ventricular aneurysm
- Recurrent arrhythmias

DRESSLER SYNDROME

D ressler syndrome is the late pericarditis occurring 1-8 weeks after acute MI. It is seen rarely and exact pathogenesis is unknown but autoimmune mechanism has been suggested.

It is characterized by chest discomfort, pleuritic chest pain, arthralgia, malaise, fever, pericardial friction rub, elevated TLC and ESR.

ECG shows ST elevation with concavity upwards or saddle-shaped diffuse ST elevations &/or PR depression.

Echocardiography may show pericardial effusion.

Treatment is the same as for the early post-MI pericarditis. Aspirin or other NSAIDs may be given. Corticosteroids can be considered in resistant cases and colchicine to prevent recurrence.

NEW YORK HEART ASSOCIATION (NYHA) CLASSIFICATION OF HEART FAILURE

- **Class I:** No limitation of physical activity.
- **Class II:** Slight limitation of physical activity, in which ordinary physical activity leads to fatigue, palpitation, or dyspnea; the person is comfortable at rest
- **Class III:** Marked limitation of physical activity, in which less-than-ordinary activity results in fatigue, palpitation, or dyspnea; the person is comfortable at rest.
- **Class IV:** Inability to carry on any physical activity without discomfort but also symptoms of heart failure at rest, with increased discomfort if any physical activity is undertaken.

LAND-MARK TRIALS

. ISIS-1

International Study of Infarct Survival-1

This was the first study which showed the benefit of treatment (β-blocker) in acute MI. Before this study it was thought that mortality of acute MI can't be influenced by any treatment.

In this RCT 16,027 patients with acute MI were randomly given β-blocker (atenolol 5-10 mg IV over 5 min followed by 100 mg PO daily for 7 days). The mortality was observed in the first week and longer follow-up for 20 months.

There was significant reduction in the vascular deaths in atenolol group. With greater benefit on day 1 due to reduction of acute myocardial rupture. Further reduction in deaths was observed after 1 year.

Ref: Lancet 1986; ii:57-66.

◆ ISIS-2

> This study showed the benefit of using the anti-platelet aspirin and thrombolytic SK in acute MI.

In this RCT, 17,187 patients with acute MI were randomized to IV SK, oral aspirin either alone or in combination and placebo and followed up to 34 months.

There was significant reduction in 5 week mortality with SK alone, aspirin alone, or in combination.

SK was associated with more bleeds requiring blood transfusion but fewer strokes. Aspirin significantly reduced the non-fatal re-infarcts and non-fatal stroke.

Ref: Lancet 1988; ii:349-60.

◆ ISIS-3

> This study compared the three thrombolytic agents SK, t-PA and anistreplase with aspirin or aspirin plus heparin.

In this RCT, 41,299 patients with acute MI were randomized to SK, t-PA, APSAC, plus aspirin or aspirin plus heparin and followed for 6 months.

The addition of heparin resulted in slightly fewer

deaths and more major non-cerebral bleeds but no significant increase in cerebral hemorrhage; there was no significant difference in mortality after 2 months.

APSAC group had more reports of allergy and cerebral bleeds compared to SK, with similar survival rates. In t-PA group there were more cerebral bleeds but fewer re-infarcts compared to SK, without any significant difference in mortality between the groups.

Ref: Lancet 1992; 339:753-70.

◆ ISIS-4

This study refuted the role of nitrates and magnesium in the management of acute MI.

In this RCT, 58,050 patients with acute MI were randomly given oral nitrate, captopril, or IV magnesium, separately or in combination in addition to standard therapy and followed for 5 weeks.

In contrast to magnesium and nitrate, the captopril group had a small but significant survival benefit that was maintained after I year, with greatest benefit in those with highest risk.

Ref: Lancet 1995; 345:669-85.

◆ GISSI-1

Gruppo Italiano per lo Studio della Strepto-chinasinell Infarto miocardio

> This study proved the benefit of the early use of thrombolytic therapy in acute MI.

In this RCT 11521 patients with acute MI were randomized to get SK and followed-up for 1 year.

At 21 days there was significant reduction in mortality in the SK group. However, in those treated within 3 hours the reduction in mortality was highly significant. At 12 months the relative risk reduction of total mortality was also highly significant.

Ref: Lancet 1987; ii: 871-4.

◆ GISSI-2

> This study established the advantage of TPA over SK regarding the risk of major bleeding when used for thrombolysis in acute MI.

In this RCT 12,490 patients with acute MI were randomized to get SK or TPA with and without Heparin and followed-up for 6 months.

There was no significant difference in the combined end-points of death, and severe LV damage, rates of in-hospital complications, (15 days post-thrombolysis), or rates of re-infarction in all the groups with or without heparin. Major bleeding occurred more frequently in the SK group compared to TPA.

Hypertensive patients had higher mortality through-out the follow-up period.

Ref: J Hypertens 1996; 14:743-50.

◆ GISSI-3

> This study established the use of ACE-Is in acute MI and that nitrates have no role in the management of AMI.

In this RCT, 18,895 patients presenting within 24 hours of symptoms of acute MI were randomized to receive li-sinopril, nitrates, or neither of these as controls and followed for 6 months.

Lisinopril significantly reduced the overall mortality and LV dysfunction while nitrates had no influence on the outcome.

Ref: Am Coll Cardiol 1996; 27:37-44.

◆ GISSI-PREVENZIONE

This study proved the benefit of polyunsaturated fatty acids (PUFA) in the diet to prevent CV deaths.

In this RCT 11,324 patients within 3 months of MI were randomized to dietary supplements PUFA and vitamin E and followed for 3.5 years. The patients had concomitant therapy with aspirin, β-blockers and ACE-I.

Vitamin E had no impact upon the risk of death, non-fatal MI or non-fatal stroke, but there was significant reduction in these end-points with PUFA.

Ref: Lancet 1999; 354:447-53.

◆ DIGAMI

Diabetes Insulin & Glucose infusion in Acute MI

This study established that insulin-glucose infusion followed by multidose insulin therapy improved the long-term survival in diabetic patients after acute MI.

In this study, 620 patients with suspected MI and blood glucose >11 mmol/l on admission were randomized to continuous IV insulin infusion for 24 hours followed by SC insulin for 3 months versus conventional therapy. Mean Follow-up 1 year (3.4 years for second, and 7.3 years for third report)

The insulin-glucose treated patients had lower 1-year

mortality. Mortality reduction was most significant in patients with low CV risk profile or no previous insulin therapy.

At 3.4 years, the mortality reduction associated with insulin was maintained.

At 7.3 years, 89% patients died in intensive glycemic control group vs 91% in control group.

The median survival was 7 years in intensive glycemic control group vs. 4.7 years in control group.

Ref: J Am Coll Cardiol. 1995; 26:57-65.
BMJ. 1997; 314:1512-5.

◆ SAVE
Survival and Ventricular Enlargement

This study showed that ACE-Is reduce the mortality from CV causes after MI with LV dysfunction and should be prescribed for post-MI patients with asymptomatic LV dysfunction.

In this RCT, 2231 patients with EF ≤40% but without overt heart failure within 3-16 days post-MI were randomly assigned to receive captopril or placebo and followed for 42 months.

Significant risk reduction was found among captopril: death (all causes), CV death, MI. Captopril group experienced lower rates of hospitalization due to heart failure and recurrent MI.

Ref: N Eng J Med 1992; 327:669-77.

Herz. 1993; 18 Suppl 1:430-5.

◆ HOPE
Heart Outcomes Prevention Evaluation

> This study showed that ACE-Is significantly reduce the CV events including MI, stroke and death in high-risk patients even in the absence of LV dysfunction.

In this study, 9297 patients at high risk of future fatal or non-fatal CV events by virtue of age >55 years, existing or previous CV disease, or diabetes (with at least one other risk factor, either known vascular disease or other factors such as smoking, high cholesterol or HT), not known to have ↓ LV EF or heart failure were randomized to receive ramipril or placebo plus vitamin E or placebo and followed for 6 years. The concomitant medication included, antihypertensive drugs (excluding ACE-I), lipid-lowering agents or aspirin.

The trial was stopped 6 months early on advice of Data Monitoring Committee because of convincing evidence of benefit of ramipril on combined primary endpoint of CV death, non-fatal MI and non-fatal stroke.

The results in 3,577 diabetic subjects were even more striking, with reduction in combined endpoints and in particular the reduction in MI far exceeded that which would be expected from the modest fall in BP.

In vitamin E group there was no significant difference in the primary or secondary end-points.

Ref: N Engl J Med. 2000.

CHOLESTEROL TRIALS

The studies have proved the CV benefits of lipid-lowering therapy. In fact, the studies have established that lipid lowering therapy should target the high-risk groups for CV events rather than depending merely upon the cholesterol level of the individual. Studies on primary and secondary prevention are grouped separately.

PRIMARY PREVENTION

• WOSCOPS

West of Scotland Coronary Prevention Study

This study showed the benefit of treating healthy hypercholesterolemic men who were at high risk of developing CV heart disease in the future.

In this RCT 6,595 men aged 45-64 years with LDL cholesterol 4-6 mmol/L and no history of MI were randomized to receive pravastatin 40 mg or placebo and followed for 5 years.

TC and LDL-C were significantly lowered and there was relative risk reduction in the number of definite coronary events and in non-fatal MI, death from all CV causes and all-cause mortality.

Ref: Eur Heart J 1996; 17:163-4.

• AFCAPS /TEXCAPS

Air Force/Texas Coronary Atherosclerosis Prevention Study

This study showed that lipid lowering therapy can reduce the CV events in primary prevention of patients with normal cholesterol levels.

In this RCT, 5608 men and 997 women with normal or mildly elevated TC, or LDL-C, low HDL-C and no clinically evident atherosclerotic disease were randomized to receive lovastatin 20-40 mg daily or placebo and followed for 5.2 years.

Lovastatin significantly reduced LDL-C and increased HDL-C. The incidence of first major acute coronary events, MI, unstable angina, or coronary re-vascularization were significantly reduced.

Ref: Am J Cardiol 2001. JAMA 1999; 281:414-9.

SECONDARY PREVENTION
◆ **4S**

Scandinavian Simvastatin Survival Study

> This study established the importance of treating hypercholesterolemic patients with established CV heart disease.

In this RCT 4,444 patients age 35-69 years with TC 5.5-8.0 mmol/L (after 8 weeks of dietary therapy) were randomized to 20 mg simvastatin or placebo and followed for 5.4 years.

There was relative risk reduction in all-cause mortality, coronary mortality, coronary events, cost of hospitalization, and re-vascularization procedures in simvastatin group. Simvastatin significantly reduced the risk of major coronary events in all quartiles of baseline TC, LDL and HDL cholesterol to a comparable degree in each quartile.

Ref: Eur Heart 1996; 17:1001-7.

◆ CARE

Cholesterol and Recurrent Events

> This study proved the benefit of treating patients with myocardial ischemia and cholesterol levels within normal limits.

In this RCT 4,159 patients aged 21-75 years having MI 3-20 months before inclusion with TC <240 mg/dl, LDL-C 115-274 mg/dl, triglycerides <350 mg/dl and followed for 5 years.

The pravastatin group had lower risk of fatal and non-fatal MI, CABG, and PTCA.

There was no reduction in coronary events if baseline TC was <125 mg/dl. The reduction in coronary events with statin therapy was greater in women and patients with higher pre-treatment levels of cholesterol.

Ref: N Engl J Med 1996; 335:1001-9.

◆ LIPID

Long-term Intervention with Pravastatin in Ischemic Disease

> This study showed the benefit of pravastatin therapy in patients with CHD with a range of initial cholesterol levels.

In this RCT 9,014 patients aged 31-75 years with a history of MI or hospitalization for unstable angina and initial plasma TC 155-271 mg/dl were randomized to receive pravastatin 40 mg daily or placebo and followed for 6.1 years. Both groups received advice on following a cholesterol-lowering diet.

Ref: N Engl J Med 1998; 339:1349-57.

◆ MIRACL
Myocardial Ischemia Reduction with Aggressive Cholesterol Lowering

> This study showed that lipid lowering therapy is useful in the setting of ACS.

In this RCT 3,086 patients were randomized to receive atorvastatin 80 mg daily initiated 24-96 hours after ACS or placebo for 16 weeks.

There was no significant difference in the risk of death, non-fatal MI, or cardiac arrest between the two groups. However atorvastatin group had a lower risk of recurrent ischemic events requiring hospitalization.

Ref: JAMA 2001; 285:1711-8.

◆ AVERT
Atorvastatin Versus Revascularisation Treatment

> This study showed the superiority of aggressive lipid lowering therapy over PTCA in patients with low risk mild to moderate stable CAD.

Treatment with atorvastatin significantly reduced LDL-C levels, and was associated with significant reduction in ischemic events and delay in time to first ischemic event.

Ref: Can J Cardiol 2000; 16:11A-3A.

◆ HPS
Heart Protection Study

> This study demonstrated the benefits of cholesterol-lowering statin therapy in patients with PAD, regardless of the presenting cholesterol levels and other presenting features.

More than 20,000 UK adults; 6748 with PAD and 13,788 other high-risk participants were randomly allocated to receive 40 mg simvastatin or placebo, yielding an average LDL cholesterol difference of 1.0 mmol/l and followed for 5 years.

For participants with PAD, simvastatin was associated with a highly significant relative reduction in the rate of first major vascular event.

Overall, among all participants, there was significant relative reduction in the rate of first peripheral vascular event, irrespective of baseline LDL-C and other factors.

Ref: J Vasc Surg 2007; 45:645-5.

SYSTEMIC LUPUS ERYTHEMATOSUS

Multi-system disorders have more chances to appear in the exams and SLE is a good example of such a disease. Lupus nephritis is the most serious manifestation of this disease.

The summary and management plan of a typical case of SLE is given below:

SUMMARY

This lady Mrs. Batool, 45 years old, from Multan, presented with shortness of breath and chest pain on the left side, aggravated by taking deep breath and by coughing. She is married for more than 20 years with no live issues; initially she had two abortions and after that she has not conceived for a long time.

On examination she has got a butterfly rash on her face, Pule is 72 beats/min, regular, and BP 170/105 mmHg (without medications). Chest examination revealed dull percussion note on the left lower zone with diminished vocal fremitus, vocal resonance and breath sounds.

Heart, abdomen, and CNS examination are unremarkable.

My provisional diagnosis is:

SLE

She has left-sided pleural effusion and HT. In view of recurrent abortions she might have anti-phospholipid syndrome.

MANAGEMENT PLAN

I will work-out to confirm the diagnosis of SLE using the American College of Rheumatology criteria.

I will perform certain investigations like FBC, ESR/CRP, Auto-antibody tests (including ANA, Anti-dsDNA, Anti-Phospholipid antibodies, RA factor), Urinalysis with microscopy, U&Es, Creatinine (eGFR), LFTs, ABGs, Chest x-ray, and USG of abdomen especially for kidneys.

I will prescribe anti-hypertensive agents, preferably in combination like CCB+ARB.

Pleural effusion will need investigations (Pleural fluid analysis) and corticosteroids, and other immune-modulating agents.

If investigations show renal involvement, I will refer the patient to a Nephrologist for possible renal biopsy and its specific management.

DISCUSSION

The discussion in a patient with SLE will usually revolve around the diagnostic issues and the management, especially of LN.

Other connective tissue disorders or the role of autoantibodies in the diagnosis may also be discussed in general.

SYSTEMIC LUPUS ERYTHEMATOSUS

S ystemic lupus erythematosus is a relapsing and remitting, autoimmune, inflammatory disorder, with diverse manifestations, ranging from mild rash or arthritis to serious involvement of the kidneys or CNS.

Its prevalence is 15 to 50 per 100,000 population. It is more common in females with a male to female ratio of 1:8.

CLINICAL FEATURES

As SLE can affect almost any organ system, its presentation and course are highly variable. Classically, it presents with a triad of fever, joint pains, and rash in a young lady.

Its most serious manifestation is LN. However, patients may present with any of the following manifestations:

Constitutional: Fever, malaise, anorexia, weight loss.

Musculoskeletal: Arthralgia, arthritis, myalgia, avascular necrosis of bones.

Dermatologic: Malar rash, photosensitivity, discoid rash, oral ulceration.

Renal: Acute nephritis, acute or chronic renal failure.

Neuropsychiatric: Seizures, psychosis.

Pulmonary: Pleurisy, pleural effusion, pneumonitis, interstitial lung disease, PAH.

GI: Nausea, dyspepsia, abdominal pain.

Hepatic: Autoimmune hepatitis, chronic active hepatitis, granulomatous hepatitis.

Cardiac: Pericarditis, myocarditis.

Hematologic: Leukopenia, lymphopenia, anemia, thrombocytopenia.

INVESTIGATIONS

- FBC, U&Es, Creatinine, Urinalysis with microscopy, ESR/CRP, LFTs, CK, spot protein/creatinine ratio, autoantibody tests including ANA & anti-DsDNA, Complement levels.
- X-rays of affected joints, Chest x-ray & CT, echocardiography, MRI/MRA of brain, Cardiac MRI.
- Renal biopsy, arthrocentesis, LP or skin biopsy for immunoflourescent staining in selected patients.

DIAGNOSIS

SLE is diagnosed on the basis of the ACR criteria. Systemic Lupus International Collaborating Clinics (SLICC) group has revised and validated the ACR criteria. They classify a person as having SLE in the presence of biopsy-proven LN and positive ANA or anti-dsDNA or if 4 of the 11 diagnostic criteria (at least one clinical and one immunologic) are present.

Four of the 11 ACR diagnostic criteria have a sensitivity of 85% and specificity of 95% for the diagnosis of SLE.

MNEMONIC FOR ACR DIAGNOSTIC CRITERIA OF SLE

SOAP	BRAIN	MD
1. Serositis 2. Oral ulcers 3. Arthritis 4. Photo-sensitivity	5. Blood disorders 6. Renal involvement 7. ANA 8. Immunologic phenomena 9. Neurologic disorder	10. Malar rash 11. Discoid rash

Key: ACR - American College of Rheumatology, SLE - Systemic lupus erythematosus, ANA - Anti-nuclear antibodies.

MANAGEMENT

Various agents are used in the treatment of SLE depending upon the severity and extent of disease.

- HCQ
- Corticosteroids
- Non-biologic DMARDs:

CYC, MTX, AZA, MMF, Cyclosporine
- NSAIDs
- Biologic DMARDs: Belimumab, Rituximab, IV immunoglobulins

PROGNOSIS

Five-year survival rate for SLE is >90%, and 10-year survival rate >80%.

The leading causes of morbidity and mortality are: infection, renal failure, neurologic and cerebrovascular events (thrombotic complications).

AUTO-ANTIBODIES ASSOCIATED WITH SLE

ANA: Sensitive but not specific. Present in 90-99% cases; homogenous or speckled.

Anti-dsDNA: Specific (70-95%) but not sensitive. Associated with LN, and vasculitis; titre may parallel the disease activity especially in LN.

Anti-Ro: Associated with Sjogren/SLE

overlap. Present in 15-35% cases.

Anti-La: Associated with neonatal lupus, photosensitivity, subacute cutaneous lupus. Present in anti-Ro positive cases with negative ANA.

Anti-Sm (anti-Smith): Very specific for SLE. Present in 30% cases.

Anti-U1-RNP: Associated with MCTD, Raynaud's. Uncommon with nephritis. Present in 40% cases.

Anti-histone: Present in 90% cases of DLE and in 0-60% cases in SLE. Mild arthritis and ostitis.

Anti-phospholipid antibodies: About 10% SLE patients may have anti-phospholipid syndrome, which is characterized by thrombosis and recurrent abortions.

LUPUS NEPHRITIS

L upus nephritis (LN) is the most serious manifestation of SLE. Clinically evident LN occurs in 50-60% of patients with SLE. Its management depends upon the class of disease, although all varieties get benefitted from HCQ.

Class I - Minimal change: Presents with normal urinalysis and serum creatinine.

No specific treatment required.

Class II - Mesangial proliferative: Presents with microscopic hematuria /proteinuria.

No specific treatment, ACE-I for HT.

Class III - Focal proliferative: Hematuria /proteinuria $\pm$ HT, ↓ GFR $\pm$ Nephrotic syndrome.

ACE-I for HT. Induce with steroids + MMF or CYC. Maintenance with MMF or AZA.

Class IV - Diffuse proliferative:

Hematuria /proteinuria, HT, ↓ GFR $\pm$ Nephrotic. syndrome.

Treatment as for class III.

Class V - Membranous: Proteinurea leading to

nephrotic syndrome.

ACE-I for HT. If nephrotic range proteinuria, induce with MMF + Steroids. Maintenance with MMF or AZA.

Class VI - Advanced sclerotic: ESRD.

Treatment is RRT.

DRUG-INDUCED LUPUS

D rug-induced lupus (DILE) is an idiosyncratic reaction to certain drugs. Usually presents in old
age and is uncommon in blacks.

The disease is generally mild with arthritis, serositis,
and skin manifestations. Renal and CNS involvement is
not frequent.

Anti-histone antibodies are present in 95% of cases and
complement levels are normal. Anti-DNA antibodies are
absent

The disease usually reverses in 4–6 weeks-time after
stopping the offending drug.

The commonly implicated drugs are:

- Procainamide
- Hydralazine
- Penicillamine
- Minocycline
- Isoniazid (INH)
- Interferon
- Methyldopa
- Quinidine
- Chlorpromazine
- Diltiazem
- Anti-TNF (esp. Infliximab)

DISCOID LUPUS

Discoid lupus erythematosus (DLE) is the mild form of disease that gets its name from the coin-shaped skin lesions.

Women of 20 to 40 years age may have a higher risk.

Aggravating factors include stress, infection, and trauma.

It causes a severe rash that tends to get worse when exposed to sunlight. It can appear anywhere on the body, but mostly on the scalp, neck, hands, and feet. Severe cases can lead to permanent scarring, hyperpigmentation, and hair loss.

Skin biopsy is usually required for diagnosis. Early treatment can help to prevent permanent scarring.

Sun-protective measures like sunscreens, photo-protective clothing, wide-brimmed hats and behavior alteration is mandatory. Give vitamin D supplements to avoid deficiency.

Standard medical therapy includes topical or intralesional corticosteroids and HCQ. Topical calcineurin inhibitors have also been used.

Systemic corticosteroids are typically avoided because of the need for prolonged use and expected side-effects.

For recalcitrant disease, immunosuppressants and immunomodulators, like MTX, MMF, AZA should be considered.

For scarring and pigment changes, filler, laser technology, and plastic surgery may be options.

About 5% people with discoid lupus will develop SLE at some point.

PSYCHOSIS IN SLE

P sychosis is a rare but well-established manifestation of SLE and it can also occur with high dose corticosteroids. If a patient with SLE on high dose steroids develops psychosis, it poses a diagnostic dilemma. No single clinical, laboratory, neuropsychological, or imaging test can differentiate between the two.

However, there are certain points in favor of each: Steroid psychosis usually occurs with high doses and in the first 1-2 weeks after starting it and resolves after its discontinuation.

Hallucinations are usually auditory in steroid psychosis and visual in lupus psychosis.

Lupus psychosis may be associated with anti-P antibodies and reduced levels of C3 & C4 in the CSF.

LAND-MARK TRIALS

Lupus nephritis is the most serious complication of SLE that occurs in 50-60% of patients and is associated with significant morbidity and mortality. If we look back on the history of treatment of LN, we see that relatively recent advances in the knowledge about its pathophysiology have revolutionized its treatment and improved the survival.

◆ Lupus nephritis study

This was one of the first studies to describe LN using kidney biopsy and to classify it on the histologic basis. It showed the benefit of using steroids in LN.

In this study, 74 patients with LN were described clically and pathologically using renal biopsy (light, electron and immunofluorescent microscopy) and treated the most active (diffuse) GN with high or low dose steroids and followed for 5 years.

Patients who received steroids survived longer, and high dose showed a survival advantage over the low dose.

Ref: Q J Med 1983; 52:311-31.

◆ NIH study

> This study showed that high dose steroid therapy alone was inferior to cytotoxic regimen.

In this study, 107 patients with active LN were given steroids plus AZA, oral or IV CYC, or a combination and were followed for seven years.

The results reached statistical significance for reducing the risk of ESRD for IV CYC versus prednisone alone.

Ref: N Engl J Med 1986; 314:614-9.

◆ MMF study

> This study demonstrated that induction with MMF plus prednisolone (regime with lesser side-effects) was as effective as CYC plus prednisolone.

In this study, 42 patients with diffuse proliferative LN were either given prednisolone and MMF for 12 months or prednisolone and CYC for 6 months, followed by prednisolone and AZA for 6 months.

MMF and prednisolone was as effective as a regimen of CYC and prednisolone followed by AZA and prednisolone with lesser side effects.

Ref: N Engl J Med 2000; 343:1156-62.

◆ MAINTAIN

> This study showed that MMF was non-significantly better than AZA in the maintenance therapy for LN.

In this study, 105 patients with proliferative LN were included by IV CYC and steroids. At week 12 they were randomized to MMF or AZA as maintenance therapy and followed for 48 months.

Fewer renal flares were observed in patients receiving MMF but the difference did not reach statistical significance.

Ref: Ann Rheum Dis 2010; 69:2083–9.

◆ ELNT
Euro Lupus Nephritis Trial

> This study showed that low and high dose CYC were associated with comparable outcomes.

In this trial, 90 SLE patients with proliferative GN were randomly assigned to high-dose IV CYC regimen or low-dose IV CYC regimen, each followed by AZA and followed for 41 months.
Low and high dose CYC had comparable outcomes.

Ref: Arthritis Rheum 2002; 46:2121-31.

◆ ALMS
Aspreva Lupus Management Study

> This study established the efficacy of MMF to IV CYC for induction and that MMF was superior than AZA in maintenance therapy.

In this RCT, 370 patients with biopsy-proven active LN were randomized to either MMF or CYC and assessed at 24 weeks. All patients had oral prednisone 60 mg/day with as per protocol taper.

MMF and IV CYC had similar effect in induction treatment. There was better response to MMF in Blacks and Hispanics

Patients who met renal response criteria at 24 weeks were subsequently re-randomized to either MMF or AZA as maintenance therapy.

MMF was superior to AZA in maintaining renal response and preventing relapse.

Ref: J Am Soc Nephrol 2009; 20:1103–12.

◆ BLISS-52
Belimumab in Subjects with SLE-52

> This was the first study which proved the efficacy and safety of biological treatment in SLE.

In this RCT, 867 patients with active SLE were randomly assigned to belimumab 1 mg/kg, 10 mg/kg, or placebo by IVI on days 0, 14, 28, and then every 28 days, with standard of care and followed for 52 weeks.

Significantly higher SLE Responder Index (SRI) rates were noted with belimumab.

Ref: Lancet 2011; 377:721–31.

◆ BLISS-76
Belimumab in Subjects with SLE-76

> This study showed that belimumab 10 mg/kg plus standard therapy significantly reduced the disease activity and severe flares in SLE and was generally well-tolerated.

In this RCT, 819 moderate to severe seropositive SLE patients were randomized to 1 mg/kg belimumab, 10 mg/kg, or placebo on days 0, 14, 28 and then every 28 days for further 72 weeks.

Belimumab 10 mg/kg plus standard therapy met the primary efficacy end-point, generating a significantly greater SRI response compared to placebo.

Serious and severe adverse events, including infections, laboratory abnormalities, malignancies, and deaths, were comparable across groups.

Ref: Arthritis Rheum 2011; 63:3918–30.

◆ TAC vs. MMF

> This study showed that TAC was non-inferior to MMF

when combined with prednisolone for induction therapy in LN.

In this RCT, 150 SLE patients with biopsy-proven active LN were randomized to TAC or MMF for induction and followed for 6 months. All patients had prednisolone for 6 weeks then forced taper per protocol to <10 mg/day.

After 6 months, the therapy was changed to AZA maintenance, while non-responders were treated with salvage CYC and glucocorticoids and followed-for 5 years.

There was no difference in proportion of patients meeting the primary endpoint with complete renal response. The need for salvage CYC treatment was also similar between the groups.

With long-term maintenance with AZA, a non-significant trend of higher incidence of renal flares and renal function decline was observed with TAC regimen.

Ref: Annals Rheumatic Dis 2016; 75:30–6.

MULTIPLE SCLEROSIS

Multiple sclerosis (MS), although not a common disease is quite frequently shown in the exams. Although it is a rare disease in the Asia but not so in the Western word.

SUMMARY

This lady, Miss Bhitanni 38 years old, unmarried, from Jandola, presented with weakness of both her lower limbs and difficulty in walking due to weakness and clumsiness.

Five years ago she had loss of vision in her right eye which recovered after two weeks therapy (including high dose steroids) prescribed by the ophthalmologist.

On examination she has got spastic paraparesis, internuclear ophthalmoplegia and cerebellar signs demonstrable in the upper limbs.

Ophthalmoscopy revealed right optic atrophy.

My provisional diagnosis is:

Multiple Sclerosis

MANAGEMENT PLAN

I will perform her MRI of the brain and spinal cord to check for "demyelination", CSF examination for "oligoclonal bands", and neurophysiologic study for "evoked potentials" to reach the diagnosis employing the McDonald criteria (revised 2017).

I will also perform baseline investigations like FBC, Blood sugar, U&Es, and urinalysis.

I will refer the patient to a Neurologist for further assessment and management. After establishing the diagnosis, the patient can be managed at home.

Initially, for acute episode the patient will need high dose parenteral corticosteroids (Methyl Prednisolone 300 mg IVI for 3 days) to abort the acute episode or relapse and later mainly the immunomodulatory / immunosuppressive therapy and supportive & symptomatic therapy.

I will specifically address her social and occupational needs, and provide her active physiotherapy and rehabilitation facilities.

I would like to involve her GP in the long-term management and a specialist appointment at 4 weeks after his discharge from the hospital.

DISCUSSION

Discussion will move around the diagnostic and management issues. Some hints for the proper answers of the possible questions are given below.

MULTIPLE SCLEROSIS

Multiple sclerosis (MS) is a demyelinating disease of unknown etiology, characterized by acute episodes of neurologic deficits, at various places in the nervous system, with spontaneous but partial remissions and relapses.

Its precise cause is not known but indirect evidence supports an autoimmune etiology, likely triggered by an environmental exposure in a genetically susceptible host.

It is more common in the females, with a male to female ratio of 1:2.

MS occurs worldwide but its prevalence varies widely. It is a rare disease in the Asia but not so in the Western countries.

PATHOLOGY

There is an immune-mediated inflammatory reaction that attacks the myelinated axons in the CNS, destroying the myelin sheath and axons in a variable degree producing significant physical disability within 20-25 years in >30% of patients.

MS derives its name from the multiple scars visible macroscopically on the brain. These lesions are termed as "plaques". Plaques are 2-10 mm in size, well-demarcated, grey or pink areas distinguished from the surrounding white matter. These are areas with chronic inflammation, demyelination and gliosis.

There is predilection for distinct sites in the brain and spinal cord:

- Optic nerves

- Periventricular region

- Brain stem and its cerebellar connections

- Cervical spinal cord: Corticospinal tracts and poster-

   ior column

CLINICAL FEATURES

The hallmark of MS is symptomatic episodes of CNS involvement that are "separated in time and space" i.e. occur months or years apart and affect the different anatomic locations. The duration of attack should be longer than 24 hours.

Types:

- Relapsing-remitting MS (RRMS)   85-90%
- Primary progressive MS (PPMS)   10-15%
- Progressive relapsing MS (PRMS)   (<5%)
- Secondary progressive MS (SPMS)   (75% of RRMS develop into SPMS in 35 years).

Characteristic presentation: Depends upon the area affected.

- **Optic neuritis:** The most common early presentation. There is blurring or loss of vision (or loss of color vision) in one eye.

Most cases of optic neuritis are retrobulbar – "the patient sees nothing, and the doctor sees nothing" (i.e. the fundus is normal). Most patients develop retrobulbar pain worse with ocular movement.

Later, fundoscopy may reveal optic atrophy.

Much less commonly, patients may describe phosphenes (transient flashes of light or black squares) lasting from hours to months. Phosphenes may occur before, during or even several months after recovery.

- **Brain stem demyelination:**

VI nerve palsy

Internuclear ophthalmoplegia (INO))

Nystagmus

One-and-a-half syndrome (VI nerve palsy + INO)

- **Spinal cord lesion:** Spastic paraplegia

Uncommon presentations:

Epilepsy, trigeminal neuralgia, dementia, psychosis.

Late stage MS:

Severely disabled young adult with spastic tetraparesis, ataxia, optic atrophy, nystagmus, brainstem signs (e.g. INO), pseudobulbar palsy and incontinence of urine.

Dementia is common.

Death follows from uremia &/or bronchopneumonia.

UHTHOFF'S PHENOMENON

Exacerbation of symptoms of MS after a hot bath, exercise, or fever.

Usually there is blurring of vision in an eye previously affected by optic neuritis.

It typically reverses rapidly on restoration of euthermia.

LHERMITTES SIGN

Barbar chair sign

Electric shock-like tingling, radiating down the arms, spine or legs, provoked by neck flexion.

Due to disruption of sensory pathways in the mid cervical cord.

Common in MS but may occur in cervical spondylosis, vitamin B12 deficiency, syringomyelia, post-irradiation, or any lesion in the cervical cord.

INTERNUCLEAR OPHTHALMOPLEGIA

Internuclear ophthalmoplegia (INO) is commonly seen in patients with MS. It is really an art to elicit INO especially in the exam situation. Demonstration of INO in a professional manner impresses the examiner and confirms your competency.

It is due to the interruption of ipsilateral medial longitudinal fasciculus, resulting in:

Paralysis of adduction of ipsilateral eye on attempted horizontal gaze to the contralateral side. Plus horizontal jerk nystagmus in the contralateral abducting eye.

CAUSES

Unilateral:
- MS (young)
- Infarction (elderly)

Bilateral:
- Brain stem glioma (child)
- MS (adult)
- Myasthenis gravis can mimic the INO

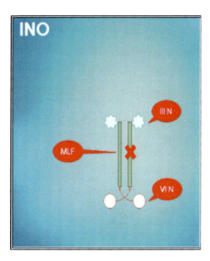

Figure 8.1: Artistic presentation of internuclear ophthalmolegia (INO).

INVESTIGATIONS

- **MRI of brain and spinal cord:** Multiple plaques of demyelination principally in the peri-ventricular region, brain stem and cervical cord.

Lesions can rarely be visible on CT scan as well.

- **Evoked potentials:** Delayed evoked potentials (visual, auditory, or somatosensory).
- **CSF examination:** Oligoclonal IgG bands in 70-90% cases.

DIAGNOSIS

MS can affect any part of the nervous system and thus can mimic any neurologic disorder.

It is diagnosed on the basis of clinical findings and supporting evidence from ancillary tests, such as MRI of brain & spinal cord, and CSF examination.

There are popular sayings in Medicine which should be kept in mind while making the diagnosis of MS.

◆ MS should not be diagnosed when all the symptoms and signs can be explained by a single lesion.

◆ MS presents with symptoms in one leg but signs in both.

McDonald criteria (Revised 2017) are employed for the diagnosis.

If the criteria are fulfilled and there is no other explanation for the clinical presentation, the diagnosis is MS.

If suspicion but the criteria are not completely fulfilled then "possible MS".

If another diagnosis arises during evaluation then the diagnosis is "not MS".

DIFFERENTIAL DIAGNOSIS

MS can mimic any neurological disorder. However the following are worth mentioning:

- Transverse myelitis
- Spinal cord neoplasm
- Spinal cord infarction
- Radiation myelitis
- Vasculitis
- Subacute combined degeneration of the cord
- Progressive multifocal leukoencephalitis
- Brain-stem glioma
- Friedreich's ataxia
- CNS sarcoidosis
- SLE
- Behcet's syndrome
- Lyme Disease
- MELAS - Mitochondrial Encephalomyopathy, Lactic Acidosis, Strokelike Episodes
- Paraneoplastic encephalomyelitis
- Acute disseminated encephalomyelitis (ADEM)

McDONALD CRITERIA FOR DIAGNOSIS
OF MULTIPLE SCLEROSIS

Clinical Presentation	Additional Data Needed for Diagnosis
■ >2 attacks ■ Objective clinical evidence of >2 lesions with reasonable historical evidence of a prior attack	None
■ >2 attacks ■ Objective clinical evidence of 1 lesion	Dissemination in space demonstrated by MRI *or* Await further clinical attack implicating a different site
■ One attack ■ Objective clinical evidence of >2 lesions	Dissemination in time demonstrated by MRI *or* second clinical attack *or* demonstration of CSF-specific oligoclonal bands
■ One attack ■ Objective clinical evidence of 1 lesion (clinically isolated syndrome)	Dissemination in space demonstrated by MRI or await a second clinical attack implicating a different CNS site and Dissemination in time, demonstrated by MRI or second clinical attack
■ Insidious neurologic pro-	One year of disease progression and dissemination

gression sug-gestive of MS	in space, demonstrated by 2 of the following: • One or more T2 lesions in brain, in regions characteristic of MS • Two or more T2 focal lesions in spinal cord • Positive CSF

Notes: An attack is defined as a neurologic disturbance of the kind seen in MS. It can be documented by subjective report or objective observation, but it must last for at least 24 hrs. Pseudo attacks and single paroxysmal episodes must be excluded. To be considered separate attacks, at least 30 days must elapse between the onset of one and another event.

MANAGEMENT
Acute episode:
- **Parenteral short course high-dose corticosteroids:**

Methyl Prednisolone 1 g IVI OD x 3 days. It hastens the recovery from acute exacerbation but doesn't influence the long-term outcome.
- **Plasmapheresis:**

Can be used for severe attacks if steroids are contraindicated or ineffective.

- **Identification and control of precipitants:**

Aggressively treat infections with antibiotics.

Normalize the body temperature with antipyretics if fever.

Urinary drainage and skin care, as appropriate.

Long-term management:
- **Immuno-modulatory Therapy:**

- Interferons: (IFN beta-1a, IFN beta-1b, Peginterferon beta-1a)

- Glatiramer acetate

- Monoclonal antibodies

- Sphingosine 1-phosphate receptor modulators: Siponimod, fingolimod, ozanimod

- Misc: Mitoxantrone, teriflunomide, dimethyl fumarate, monomethyl fumarate, cladribine

- Immunosupressants: MTX, AZA, CYC
  - **Therapies to relieve symptoms:**

Physiotherapy, social and occupational therapy has central role in the long-term management.

MS society provides helpful literature and support.

PROGNOSIS

MS is a relapsing-remitting disease in most of the cases, with variable and unpredictable course. Many patients continue to live self-sufficient, productive lives while others are gravely disabled.

It produces significant physical disability within 20-25 years in more than 30% of patients.

Straight-forward advice, tempered with reassurance of possible benign course in many cases is important.

DEVIC'S DISEASE
(Neuromyelitis optica)

A syndrome characterized by optic neuritis, usually bilateral, followed by (less frequently preceded) within hours to weeks by transverse myelitis.

It is due to demyelination affecting the optic nerves and spinal cord. It is a type of MS which is usually milder than usual.

Neuromyelitis optica can be confirmed by the presence of serum antibodies against aquaporin 4, a water channel expressed at major fluid-tissue barriers across the CNS.

LAND-MARK TRIALS

◆ ACTH IN MS

> This was the first RCT which proved the benefit of ACTH in acute exacerbation of MS.

In this study, 40 patients with unequivocal MS, who presented with an assessable new symptom or sign of less than 14 days duration showing no spontaneous improvement, were randomized to receive either ACTH or saline injections.

ACTH improved the symptoms, measured through subjective reports from patients in a follow-up interview.

Ref: Lancet 1961; 2:1120–2.

◆ MRI vs. CT Scan in MS

> This study showed superiority of MRI over CT scan in the diagnosis and monitoring of disease activity in MS.

In this study, 10 patients with MS were scanned by means of cranial CT with and without IV contrast enhancement, and by nuclear magnetic resonance (NMR).

CT captured 19 lesions (between 7x5 mm and 13x8 mm), whereas NMR captured 112 additional lesions varing in size from 4x3 to 12x7 mm and were particularly well seen in the periventricular region and brainstem. So NMR demonstrates abnormalities in MS on a scale not previously seen except at necropsy.

Ref: Lancet 1981; 2:1063–6.

◆ INTERFERON IN MS

> This study demonstrated the efficacy of interferon beta-1b in relapsing-remitting MS.

In this RCT, 327 patients with relapsing-remitting MS were randomized to interferon beta-1b or placebo.

The MRI results support the clinical results in showing a significant reduction in disease activity as measured by numbers of active scans and appearance of new lesions. In addition, there was an equally significant reduction in MRI detected burden of disease in the treatment as compared with placebo.

These results demonstrate that IFN-b has made a significant impact on the natural history of MS in these patients.

Ref: Neurology 1993; 43: 662–7.

◆COPOLYMER 1 MULTIPLE SCLEROSIS STUDY

> This study demonstrated the efficacy of glatiramer acetate in patients with relapsing-remitting MS.

In this study, 251 patients with relapsing-remitting MS were randomized to receive glatiramer acetate 20 mg by daily SC inj or placebo. After 35 months, 208 patients chose to continue in an open-label study with all patients receiving active drug. The patients were evaluated at 6-month intervals and during suspected relapse. The data reported was from 6 years of organized evaluation, including the double-blind phase of up to 35 months and open-label phase of over 36 months.

The study demonstrated sustained efficacy of glatiramer acetate in reducing the relapse rate and in slowing the accumulation of disability.

Ref: Mult Scler 2000; 6:255-66.

◆ TOPIC

> This study showed that treatment of clinically isolated syndrome with Teriflunomide delays conversion to MS.

In this multicentre RCT, 618 patients with the first

acute or subacute well-defined neurologic event consistent with demyelination were randomized to teriflunomide 14 mg or 7 mg per day or placebo and followed for 2 years.

Patients receiving 14 mg teriflunomide experienced 43% reduction in the risk for conversion to clinically definite MS compared with placebo. Patients who received 7 mg of the drug per day had a 37% reduction in the risk for conversion vs placebo.

Ref: http://www.medscape.com/viewarticle/803177.

BIBLIOGRAPHY

1. Papadakis MA, et al. Current Medical Diagnosis and Treatment. 2015. Lange McGraw Hill Education.
2. Keith N, et al. Some different types of essential hypertension: their course and prognosis. Am J Med Sci 1939; 196:332–9.
3. Henderson AD, et al. Hypertension-related eye abnormalities and the risk of stroke. Rev Neurol Dis 2011; 8:1–9.
4. Medscape. e-medicine. www.medscape.com
5. Mayo Clinic. Diabetic retinopathy. http://www.mayoclinic.org/diseases-conditions/diabetic-retinopathy/expert-answers/con-20023311
6. WHO. Definition and diagnosis of diabetes mellitus and intermediate hyperglycemia: Report of a WHO/IDF Consultation. http://www.who.int/diabetes/publications/Definition%20and%20diagnosis%20of%20diabetes_new.pdf
7. Wiesner, et al. United Network for Organ Sharing Liver Disease Severity Score Committee. Model for end-stage liver disease (MELD) and allocation of donor livers. Gastroenterology 2003; 124:91-6.
8. Nau KC, et al. Glycemic control in hospital-

ized patients not in intensive care: beyond sliding-scale insulin. Am Fam Physician 2010; 81:1130-5.

9. British National Formulary. BNF 79; March 2020.

10. Rimm R, et al. Overt psychopathology in systemic lupus erythematosus. Scand J Rheumatol 1988; 17:143-6.

11. Monov S, et al. Classification criteria for neuropsychiatric systemic lupus erythematosus: do they need a discussion? Hippokratia 2008; 12:103-7.

12. Lewis DA, et al. Steroid-induced psychiatric syndromes. A report of 14 cases and a review of the literature. J Affect Disord 1983; 5:319-32.

13. The Boston Collaborative Drug Surveillance Program. Acute adverse reactions to prednisone in relation to dosage. Clin Pharmacol Ther 1972; 13:694–8.

14. Hall RC, et al. Presentation of the steroid psychoses. J Nerv Ment Dis 1979; 167:229–36.

15. Powers WJ, et al. Guidelines for the early management of patients with acute ischemic stroke: 2019 Update to the 2018 guidelines for the early management of acute ischemic stroke: a guideline for healthcare professionals from the American Heart Association /American Stroke Association. Stroke 2019 Dec; 50: e344.

16. Goyal M, et al; HERMES Collaborators. Endovascular thrombectomy after large-vessel ischemic stroke: a meta-analysis of individual patient data from five randomized trials. Lancet 2016; 387:1723–31.

17. Intercollegiate Stroke Working Party. National

Clinical Guideline for Stroke, 5th Edn. London: Royal College of Physicians, 2016.

18. Lane DA, et al. Use of the CHA(2)DS(2)-VASc and HAS-BLED scores to aid decision making for thromboprophylaxis in nonvalvular atrial fibrillation. Circulation 2012; 126:860-5.

19. American Heart Association (AHA) guidelines.

20. European Society of Cardiology guidelines.

21. Marriott's Practical Electrocardiography. 12th Edn.

22. Manual of Cardiovascular Medicine. 5th Edn.

23. NICE Clinical Guidelines 2017.

24. European Association for the Study of the Liver. EASL clinical practice guidelines for the management of patients with decompensated cirrhosis. J Hepatol. 2018; 69:406–60. doi: 10.1016/j.jhep.2018.03.024

25. Aithal GP, et al. Guidelines on the management of ascites in cirrhosis. Gut. 2021; 70:9–29. doi: 10.1136/gutjnl-2020-321790

26. Biggins SW, et al. Diagnosis, evaluation, and management of ascites, spontaneous bacterial peritonitisand hepatorenal syndrome: 2021 Practice Guidance by the American Association for the study of liver diseases. 2021; Hepatology 74:1014-48. doi: 10.1002/hep.31884

27. Marrero JA, et al. Diagnosis, staging, and management of hepatocellular carcinoma: 2018 Practice Guidance by the American Association for the Study of Liver Diseases. Hepatology 2018; 68:723-50. doi: 10.1002/hep.29913

28. Garcia-Tsao, et al. Portal Hypertensive Bleeding in Cirrhosis: Risk Stratification, Diagnosis, and

Management: 2016 Practice Guidance by the American Association for the Study of Liver Diseases. Hepatology 2017; 65: 310-35. doi: 10.1002/hep.28906

29. Dasse KD, et al. Chemoembolism with drug-eluting beads for the treatment of hepato-cellular carcinoma. J Adv Pract Oncol 2016; 7:764-78.

ACKNOWLEDGEMENT

First of all I praise the almighty Allah for giving me the will and power to share my knowledge with my medical community and then I gratefully acknowledge the hard work by all the contributors, coauthors, reviewers, editorial assistants, and printers, in turning this dream into a reality.

I am especially thankful to the Amazon's "Kindle Direct Publishing" (KDP) to accommodate and globally project my work as an author, editor and a self-publisher.

I also acknowledge the Chandler Boltof Self-Publishing School from whom I took lot of online guidance while publishing this book.

ABOUT THE AUTHOR

Habibullah Khan

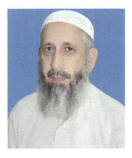

Professor Habibullah Khan, a medical graduate of Khyber Medical College, Peshawar, Pakistan session 1980; a Member of College of Physicians & Surgeons of Pakistan and a Fellow of Royal College of Physicians of Edinburgh, UK.

He worked as Professor of Medicine at Gomal Medical College, D.I.Khan. Presently working as Consultant Physician at Rauf Medical Centre, D.I.Khan.

He also served at various health sectors in the country and abroad including Army Medical Corps, Provincial Health Services, Kingdom of Saudi Arabia, and United Kingdom.

He is actively involved in research and has published more than 70 papers. During his services at GMC he initiated the research journal, "Gomal Journal of Medical Sciences" which is one of the internationally recognized and renounced medical serial today.

Made in the USA
Middletown, DE
14 January 2022

58651111R00223